HEALTHCARE ACTIVE LEARNING

HAL

GENETICS

Start date

Target completion date

Tutor for this topic

Contact number

is to

THE LEARNING CENTRE
TOWER HAMLETS COLLEGE
ARBOUR SQUARE
LONDON E1 0PS
Tel: 0171 538 5888

USING THIS WORKBOOK

The workbook is divided into 'Sessions', covering specific subjects.

In the introduction to each learning pack there is a learner profile to help you assess your current knowledge of the subjects covered in each session.

Each session has clear learning objectives. They indicate what you will be able to achieve or learn by completing that session.

Each session has a summary to remind you of the key points of the subjects covered.

Each session contains text, diagrams and learning activities that relate to the stated objectives.

It is important to complete each activity, making your own notes and writing in answers in the space provided. **Remember this is your own workbook—you are allowed to write on it.**

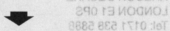

Now try an example activity.

ACTIVITY

This activity shows you what happens when cells work without oxygen. This really is a physical activity, so please only try it if you are fully fit.

First, raise one arm straight up in the air above your head, and let the other hand rest by your side. Clench both fists tightly, and then open out your fingers wide. Repeat this at the rate of once or twice a second. Try to keep clenching both fists at the same rate. Keep going for about five minutes, and record what you observe.

Stop and rest for a minute. Then try again, with the opposite arm raised this time. Again, record your observations.

Suggested timings are given for each activity. These are only a guide. You may like to note how long it took you to complete this activity, as it may help in planning the time needed for working through the sessions.

Time taken on activity

Time management is important. While we recognise that people learn at different speeds, this pack is designed to take 20 study hours (your tutor will also advise you). You should allocate time during each week for study.

Take some time now to identify likely periods that you can set aside for study during the week.

	Mon	Tues	Wed	Thurs	Fri	Sat	Sun
am							
pm							
eve							

At the end of the learning pack, there is a learning review to help you assess whether you have achieved the learning objectives.

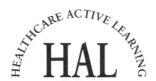

HEALTHCARE ACTIVE LEARNING

HAL

GENETICS

Patricia A. Lyne BSc PhD RGN

Reader in Nursing Research, Department of Advanced Nursing,
The North East Wales Institute

THE OPEN LEARNING FOUNDATION

CHURCHILL LIVINGSTONE

EDINBURGH LONDON MADRID MELBOURNE NEW YORK AND TOKYO 1995

CHURCHILL LIVINGSTONE
Medical Division of Longman Group UK Limited

Distributed in the United States of America by Churchill
Livingstone Inc., 650 Avenue of the Americas, New York,
N.Y. 10011, and by associated companies, branches and
representatives throughout the world.

First published 1995

ISBN 0 443 05273 5

British Library of Cataloguing in Publication Data
A catalogue record for this book is available from the
British Library.

Library of Congress Cataloging in Publication Data
A catalogue record for this book is available from the
Library of Congress

Printed and bound by Bell and Bain Ltd., Glasgow

For The Open Learning Foundation

Director of Programmes: Leslie Mapp
Series Editor: Robert Adams
Programmes Manager: Kathleen Farren
Production Manager: Steve Moulds

For Churchill Livingstone

Director (NAH): Peter Shepherd
Project Development Editor: Mairi McCubbin
Project Manager: Valerie Burgess
Design Direction: Judith Wright
Pre-press Project Manager: Neil Dickson
Pre-press Desktop Operator: Kate Walshaw
Sales Promotion Executive: Hilary Brown

The
publisher's
policy is to use
**paper manufactured
from sustainable forests**

Contents

OPEN LEARNING FOUNDATION TEAM MEMBERS

Writer: Dr Patricia A. Lyne
Reader in Nursing Research, Department of Advanced Nursing,
The North East Wales Institute

Editor: Dr Elisabeth Clarke
Distance Learning Programme Coordinator,
Royal College of Nursing

Reviewers: Professor Justus Akinsaya
Pro Vice Chancellor, International Development,
Anglia Polytechnic University

Professor John Neville
Dean, Faculty of Science and Health,
University of East London

Series Editor: Robert Adams
OLF Programme Head,
Social Work and Health and Nursing,
University of Humberside

THE OPEN LEARNING FOUNDATION

Higher education has grown considerably in recent years. As well as catering for more students, universities are facing the challenge of providing for an increasingly diverse student population. Students have a wider range of backgrounds and previous educational qualifications. There are greater numbers of mature students. There is a greater need for part-time courses and continuing education and professional development programmes.

The Open Learning Foundation helps over 20 member institutions meet this growing and diverse demand – through the production of high-quality teaching and learning materials, within a strategy of creating a framework for more flexible learning. It offers member institutions the capability to increase their range of teaching options and to cover subjects in greater breadth and depth.

It does not enrol its own students. Rather, The Open Learning Foundation, by developing and promoting the greater use of open and distance learning, enables universities and others in higher education to make study more accessible and cost-effective for individual students and for business through offering more choice and more flexible courses.

Formed in 1990, the Foundation's policy objectives are to:

- improve the quality of higher education and training

- increase the quantity of higher education and training

- raise the efficiency of higher education and training delivery.

In working to meet these objectives, The Open Learning Foundation develops new teaching and learning materials, encourages and facilitates more and better staff development, and promotes greater responsiveness to change within higher education institutions. The Foundation works in partnership with its members and other higher education bodies to develop new approaches to teaching and learning.

In developing new teaching and learning materials, the Foundation has:

- a track record of offering customers a swift and flexible response

- a national network of members able to provide local support and guidance

- the ability to draw on significant national expertise in producing and delivering open learning

- complete freedom to seek out the best writers, materials and resources to secure development.

INTRODUCTION

The science of genetics sometimes seems rather remote from everyday life and from the business of providing direct care to patients and clients. In this unit, I aim to show you that this discipline can offer valuable insights to nurses, midwives and health visitors. These insights will assist in planning and delivering high-quality care.

As a scientific discipline, genetics requires an understanding of some elaborate and sophisticated concepts and a detailed knowledge of cellular structure and function. These can only be achieved by lengthy study of the subject. They are the province of the professional geneticist. In this unit, I do not attempt to provide a watered down version of this professional training. No one would expect geneticists to deliver professional health care; similarly, health professionals are not expected to become biomedical scientists.

So rather than trying to cover the whole of the subject, I have selected four of the key concepts upon which this science is based. I have selected those concepts that are most relevant to the caring professions and which can be used to inform and improve practice. Each of the four sessions in this unit deals with one of these fundamental concepts, as follows:

Session One: Variation

This is intended to raise awareness of the differences between people, and how these can be explained. Such an understanding is essential in delivering individualised health care.

Session Two: Randomness

Many people are put off studying genetics by its numerical aspects. Session Two shows that an intelligent, professional interest in randomness is possible without any special mathematical knowledge.

Session Three: Adaptation

This part considers how people adapt to particular environments and circumstances. This concept has been influential in the development of recent theories about nursing.

Session Four: Vulnerability

Understanding how and why things go wrong involves the idea of the vulnerability of the genetic material—an idea which relates to the day-to-day concerns of all members of the nursing profession.

It may be that some of these ideas are entirely new to you. They are to very many people, and I haven't assumed that you know anything about them at this stage. This unit is intended primarily for people with no previous acquaintance with genetics.

In some ways, you could be at a disadvantage if you have studied genetics before starting this on unit. This is because I have adopted an approach which is different from the one found in standard textbooks. I have concentrated on those areas of the subject which can best inform practice in nursing, midwifery and health visiting and which will help practitioners to contribute to the current debates on the issues which arise from modern applications of this science to health care.

You may find that, even though non-technical language is used wherever possible, you need to spend quite a long time on some sections. The key genetic concepts may be challenging and unfamiliar. Please don't worry if you find that progress is slow. It is worth persevering with these concepts, because they are so important to a clear understanding of many aspects of health care.

LEARNING PROFILE

Below is a list of learning outcomes for each session in this unit. You can use it to identify your current familiarity with the subject, and so to consider how the unit can help you to develop your knowledge and understanding. The list is not intended to cover all the details discussed in every session, and so the learning profile should only be used for general guidance.

For each of the learning outcomes listed below, tick the box that corresponds most closely to your own abilities. This will provide you with an assessment of your current understanding and confidence in the areas that you will study in this unit.

	Not at all	Partly	Quite well	Very well

Session One
I can:
- explain the relevance of genetics to health-care practice ☐ ☐ ☐ ☐
- give a simple explanation of the way in which genetic and environmental factors give rise to observable differences between people ☐ ☐ ☐ ☐
- explain, in non-technical terms, the nature and origins of the genetic code ☐ ☐ ☐ ☐
- describe how the genetic code is organised into genes ☐ ☐ ☐ ☐
- give examples of the way in which the environment affects gene expression ☐ ☐ ☐ ☐
- apply these ideas to care planning. ☐ ☐ ☐ ☐

Session Two
I can:
- explain the random nature of the inheritance of gender ☐ ☐ ☐ ☐
- explain how an understanding of the role of randomness in cell division enables genetic outcomes to be predicted ☐ ☐ ☐ ☐

	Not at all	Partly	Quite well	Very well
● outline the basis of single-factor inheritance patterns	☐	☐	☐	☐
● explain how random events contribute to genetic variation	☐	☐	☐	☐
● describe the contribution of genes and the environment to the establishment of a 'normal' state	☐	☐	☐	☐
● apply these ideas to care planning.	☐	☐	☐	☐

Session Three

I can:

	Not at all	Partly	Quite well	Very well
● explain the advantages for survival of 'normal' characteristics	☐	☐	☐	☐
● give examples of survival behaviour and explain its genetic basis	☐	☐	☐	☐
● outline the effects on health of moving between environments	☐	☐	☐	☐
● make links between the concepts of adaptation and health	☐	☐	☐	☐
● suggest why characteristics may persist despite being unfavourable	☐	☐	☐	☐
● apply these ideas to health-care practice.	☐	☐	☐	☐

Session Four

I can:

	Not at all	Partly	Quite well	Very well
● summarise the causes of genetic variation	☐	☐	☐	☐
● suggest how the environment can cause genetic damage	☐	☐	☐	☐
● explain the links between random changes and ageing	☐	☐	☐	☐
● outline how genetic repair mechanisms work	☐	☐	☐	☐
● give examples of new developments in gene therapy	☐	☐	☐	☐
● apply these principles to patient care.	☐	☐	☐	☐

Variation

Introduction

Session One is divided into nine sections. Some are quite short, others are much more substantial. Each section ends at a natural break point, which will enable you to study in a series of fairly short sittings. On balance, the longer you study at one sitting, the less effectively you learn, so it is best to work for several short periods rather than one long one.

The aim of the session is to give you the opportunity to increase your awareness of the differences between people and to provide an explanation of this diversity. This understanding will contribute to your ability to plan and deliver individualised care.

I will start by asking you to make some observations about the way in which people differ, particularly within families. These will be used as the springboard for an exploration of the causes of diversity and the nature of the genetic code. The relationship between the theoretical elements and practical health care will be emphasised throughout. I will end Session One by applying the principles which have been developed to two contrasting, real-life case-studies.

Session objectives

When you have completed this session you should be able to:

- explain the relevance of genetics to health-care practice
- give a simple explanation of the way in which genetic and environmental forces give rise to the observable differences between people
- explain, in non-technical terms, the nature of the genetic code
- describe how the genetic code is organised into genes
- give examples of the way in which the environment affects gene expression
- apply these ideas to care planning.

Please note this text is written so that it can be understood by people who have not studied genetics at all in the past. It may be you have already achieved these outcomes and wish to use the material for revision purposes.

1: It runs in the family

To begin with, we will think about some of the people we meet every day and see whether the science of genetics relates to some real-life questions. Here is a description of my own family.

All three members of my immediate family are ectomorphs – two very tall, slim sons and their tall, thin father. They have slim bodies, long limbs and they never gain weight. By contrast, both I and my parents are short and stocky.

One of our sons has very striking red hair. No other living member of either family has this feature, although my nephew has reddish blond hair. Apparently, my mother had two sisters with beautiful red hair. They both died of tuberculosis in their early twenties.

My mother's surviving sister had two sons. The elder was classified as 'mentally defective', and died in an institution at the age of 16. His younger brother, born seven years later, was more fortunate. By then, more was known about the illness from which his brother had suffered. It was **phenylketonuria** (PKU) – an inherited disease for which all babies are now routinely tested at birth by means of a small blood sample taken from the heel. The younger boy had the same disease, but received treatment from birth.

When I think about my family and their characteristics, I can't help asking certain questions. For example, suppose we had a daughter. Might she have been tall and slim with red hair? Is my red-headed son, like his great aunts, likely to be susceptible to TB? What are the chances that PKU will crop up again in future generations?

These are the kinds of questions which many people ask themselves from time to time. In asking them, we are starting to explore the science of genetics.

2: Family trees

The description you have just read does not enable you to see the relationships between people in the family very clearly. A better way to do this is to draw a family tree. Geneticists have developed a particular way of doing this which is designed to make the connections as clear as possible by using a special set of conventions.

Figure 1 shows the family tree for red hair in my family, and includes an explanation of the conventions that are normally used in genetics.

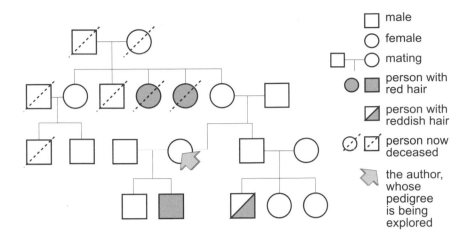

Figure 1 A family tree – or pedigree – for red hair

It would be too confusing to show more than one characteristic on a family tree, so it is usual to draw a separate diagram for each one.

Figure 2 shows the same family again, but this time it deals with PKU rather than hair colour.

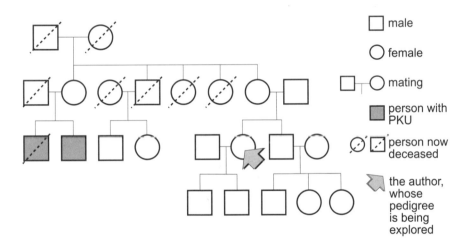

Figure 2 A family tree for PKU

ACTIVITY 1   ALLOW 20 MINUTES

Think about a family that you know well. It could be your own or someone else's – that doesn't matter, as long as you know something about at least three generations of the family. Can you identify a characteristic which has come and gone between the generations – like red hair in the family described earlier?

Write a short description of the family, and then draw a family tree to display it, using the symbols shown in *Figures 1* and *2*.

Commentary

How did you get on? Were you able to detect any characteristics that came and went between the generations?

The sorts of things that people identify when they try this exercise are usually striking physical characteristics – short legs, a prominent chin, an unusual hairline, baldness, protruding ears, strong teeth, and so on. This photograph of the Kennedy family shows several such striking physical characteristics:

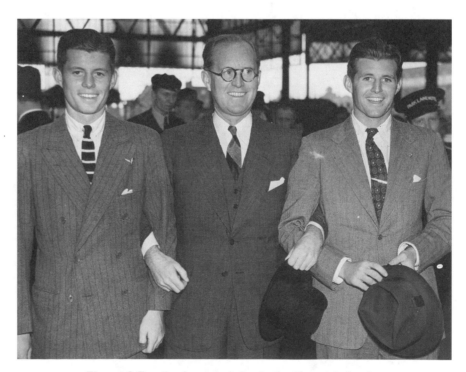

Figure 3 Family characteristics in the Kennedy family

On the other hand, the characteristics you chose might have related to abilities – physical or mental – like being musical, athletic, or good at maths. Or, they could be illnesses or disabilities.

Obviously, the larger the family, the easier it is to see patterns of inheritance in a family tree. In modern families, the numbers in each generation are usually small and the patterns don't show up too well. The family you chose may be like this, and as a consequence you may not have been able to discern any definite patterns. Nevertheless, when you return to this family tree later on, you will have an enhanced understanding of the differences which you have initially identified.

To illustrate what we can learn from a large family tree, I have provided a very well known one for the next activity. Queen Victoria and Prince Albert were the forebears of a very large family.

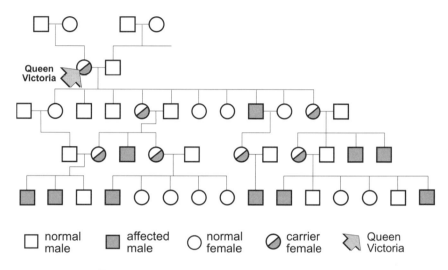

Figure 4 Part of the family tree of Queen Victoria

ACTIVITY 2

ALLOW **15** MINUTES

The characteristic shown in this Royal family tree is **haemophilia,** an inherited illness in which the blood does not clot properly and small abrasions lead to uncontrolled bleeding.

Study *Figure 4*, and note down your answers to the following questions.

1 Which is the most noticeable feature of this pattern in terms of the individuals who have been affected?

2 What do you think the link is between the affected individuals in successive generations?

3 Where do you think this inherited condition started in the Royal Family?

Commentary

While studying this family tree you may have observed that:

1 All the affected individuals are male.

2 The link between generations with an affected male is always a carrier female.

3 It is difficult, with the information provided, to be certain where the condition began. You might have guessed that it started with the Queen herself and, as we will see later, this appears to be the case.

This family tree illustrates how much can be learnt about inheritance patterns when geneticists are able to study large, well-documented families. This particular case has been very extensively studied because of the effect that this disease had on Queen Victoria's descendants. Many of these descendants later became the crowned heads of European countries.

By studying family trees and patterns of inheritance, geneticists are able to answer the kinds of question we all might ask about the characteristics that we see in families. However, for health care professionals, there are other questions which may be even more important because what we try to do is to provide individualised care. We are therefore interested in people as unique individuals.

3: Note the difference

Genetics is the science of diversity. It is to do with why living things differ and why they are similar. It involves the study of ways in which the characteristics of parents are passed on to their offspring. It is one way of explaining how any living thing comes to be the way it is at a particular time.

When a health professional makes an initial assessment of someone receiving care, they try to be aware of every aspect of that person as a unique individual in an unique situation. What the practitioner observes is the result of the many forces which have acted on that person throughout their lifetime.

Genetics provides the background we need to understand how the powerful forces of inheritance and the environment have contributed to a person's individuality. So now let's begin to look at some of the differences which are to be found in the people around us.

ACTIVITY 3

You should start this observation process by observing a group of people and considering a simple question. Look at a group of people who are all dressed in the same way – maybe you could find a photograph of a school class, or a sports team, or a party of student nurses or midwives. Or perhaps you could observe a group of your current colleagues who all wear the same uniform.

The question to consider is this:

> Does the uniform reduce or enhance the
> differences between these people?

At some time in the near future, you may like to discuss this with your colleagues, when you have a few moments to spare.

Commentary

Clearly there can be no right or wrong answer to this sort of question. It is a matter of personal opinion. For example, some people consider that wearing the same clothes exaggerates the differences between the wearers. Some individuals look good in uniform – and the colour and style seems to complement their best features. Others are not so flattered by it. In this case, the difference between them is enhanced, rather than diminished and emphasises the amazing number of ways in which the various components of a human body can be put together.

However, the way people look is only one aspect of the variation between them. The next activity gives you the opportunity to explore these variations more fully.

ACTIVITY 4

Select three people who you know well, all the same sex and about the same age. Consider the ways in which they differ from one another. In other words, select some of the characteristics that seem to vary from person to person.

The first thing which comes to mind may be their visible characteristics.

Make a list of these in Column 1 of *Table 1* (leave Column 2 until the next activity).

Next, think about how these people move, speak and generally behave.

What about their health status? Are any of the characteristics you picked up in the family tree in Activity 1 relevant? Add the characteristics to your list in Column 1.

When you have run out of ideas, stop for a few minutes and think again about the three people you chose.

Are there any subtle differences which you have missed first time round?

If so, add them to Column 1.

If you are working with other people studying this unit, you might like to combine your lists.

1. Varying characteristics	2. Source of variation

Table 1

Commentary

You may have taken a little time to get this activity under way, but it is likely that you discovered more and more characteristics as you warmed to the task.

You might have added some of the more subtle variations as a result of your second thoughts – details such as the size of ear lobes, facial symmetry, expressiveness of features, the tendency to premenstrual tension in women or the strength of beard growth in men.

You may have found it difficult to describe the characteristics you identified. This doesn't matter at all, as long as you have begun to increase your awareness of the subtlety and extent of the differences which exist, even between people of similar age and gender.

Once this awareness begins to increase, you may find yourself looking with new eyes at things you previously took for granted about the people you encounter at work and at home. And you may find yourself prompted to ask:

How does all this diversity come about, and does it serve any useful purpose?

The first part of this question forms our next topic. The second will be explored in Session Three of this unit.

4: Sources of variation

The next activity asks you to make some decisions about how the variations in the three people you studied in the previous activity came about.

ACTIVITY 5   ALLOW 5 MINUTES

For each of the characteristics you listed in the previous activity, decide on the source of the differences which you observed. Go back and list these sources in the Column 2 of *Table 1*.

For example, suppose you chose hair colour as one of the varying characteristics. Then:

- if you think the differences are solely due to factors present at birth, record the source as 'genetic'

- if, on the other hand, you feel that a person's hair colour is influenced by external factors such as the sun or the hairdresser record the source as 'environmental'

- if you feel that the colour is due to a mixture of inherited and external influences, write down 'both'. This might apply, for example, when a natural blonde has just returned from a fortnight's holiday in the Mediterranean.

Commentary

You probably found this decision easier for some characteristics than others. But on balance, as you thought it through, you will have found yourself identifying the source of much of the variation under the label 'both'. Indeed, much of the variation which we see is due to a combination of genetic and environmental influences. In many cases, it is difficult to be sure which has had the most influence.

This is a subject which has always provoked considerable discussion. It is sometimes called the **nature/nurture debate**, and remains an important issue today – as the next activity will demonstrate.

ACTIVITY 6   ALLOW **20** MINUTES

In order to emphasise the relevance of this discussion of variations, it would be useful to read the newspaper article, 'Born not made'. You will find this in the Resource Section at the end of this unit, identified as *Resource 1*. This item deals with the issue of sexual orientation and shows how the nature/nurture debate continues today.

As you read, note down what kinds of evidence the author puts forward. When you have finished, record your answers to the following questions.

1   What evidence does the author put forward to support the idea that sexual orientation is based on genetic factors?

2   What evidence does he advance in support of the view that environmental factors are more important?

3   Does the author consider that we can decide between these two points of view?

4   What relevance does this discussion have for us as health professionals?

Commentary

After reading the article, you may have been able to answer the questions along these lines.

1 The author quotes several pieces of evidence in support of a possible genetic basis for sexual orientation. These are:

   ● brain structures set up before birth
   ● pre-natal sources of childhood characteristics
   ● differences in the brain structures of people with different sexual orientation.

2 He quotes Freud's assertion that homosexuality results from parental influence.

3 He states that we do not know what makes people gay or straight, but it sounds as if he considers that the evidence for a genetic basis is stronger than that for an environmental source.

4 The title of the article – 'Born not made?' – suggests a question that we can apply to all the people we care for. We might ask ourselves whether a patient's response to health and illness is due to genetic factors, which cannot be changed, or to environmental factors, which can.

You may like to use this article as the basis for a group discussion with your colleagues on the way in which genetic and environmental factors influence the way in which variation develops, bearing in mind the kinds of evidence that can be used in the debate.

It is worth noting that the Health Section of *The Guardian* often deals with topical issues like this and may provide a good supplementary source of background reading for this unit.

I would now like to summarise the main points of the unit so far. I will do this from time to time so that you can pause and think about work that you have done. If you feel unsure about any of these points, please look back over the preceding section before you go on.

Summary of Sections 1 to 4

● We can observe a great deal of variation between people.

● What we observe is due to the interaction of genetic and environmental factors.

● The discussion about the relative contribution of these factors is relevant at the present time because of the rapid developments in genetic science which may influence all our lives.

There are still many specific situations in which we do not know how genetics and the environment interact. However, in recent years geneticists have increased our understanding of these processes dramatically. We are now going to consider what is known about the way in which inherited differences come about and how environmental influences act upon these to produce such a wide variety of different people.

5: The genetic code

What is DNA?

The variation which is present at birth, which we can identify as **genetic variation**, must have its origin in the fertilised egg at conception. This is the starting point from which every person grows. Therefore, it must contain all the information needed to make that person into a unique individual. Let us first consider the nature of that information, in order to understand how it functions.

The fertilised egg, like most other cells in the human body, contains a **nucleus**. The nucleus is a distinct region of the cell, separated from the cell contents by a membrane and acting as a control centre for the cell's activities.

Viewed through a microscope, the **nuclei** of living cells look spherical and move around inside the cells as the contents of the cells move.

Every nucleus contains substances called **nucleic acids**. These are so-called because they were first discovered in nuclei and it was thought that they did not occur anywhere else. This has since been found to be incorrect, but the name remains both as an accident of history and because they are more abundant in nuclei than in other parts of the cell.

There are two types of nucleic acid which, although constructed from similar basic materials, have different functions in the cell. Their correct chemical names are **deoxyribonucleic acid** and **ribonucleic acid**, but they are usually referred to by the abbreviations **DNA** and **RNA**.

You may well have come across DNA in your reading, or have heard it reported in the media in connection with some current controversy.

ACTIVITY 7 ALLOW 5 MINUTES

At the moment, when you hear the term DNA, what comes to mind? Make a note in the space below of the things you associate with DNA, and jot down anything which you find puzzling about it.

● Thoughts associated with DNA:

● Puzzling features:

Commentary

Many people who answer this question come up with comments such as:

'It's something to do with genetics'
'It enables cells to replicate'
'It's to do with genetic engineering, whatever that may be'
'I know it's a double helix discovered by an American, because I saw a TV play, but I've no idea what that means'
'I've heard words like cloning, fingerprinting and pre-natal diagnosis used along with it'
'It can be used to identify a child's father, can't it?'

Ideas of this kind arise from everyday experience – from the newspapers, the television and in general conversation. However, after completing this section, you will have an increased understanding of the nature of DNA and of its significance in many aspects of our lives.

DNA and the genetic code

As you made your own list, I wonder whether you added one item which is missing from the one given above. Did you make the point that *DNA carries genetic information*?

I have already introduced this idea, and will now explain it in more detail. Since this is not a course for scientists, I am not assuming that you have any understanding of chemical formulae and structures. I will therefore be using metaphors to illustrate some of the ideas that you will need to think through now.

When describing how DNA works, a useful metaphor is that of a book of instructions. We can visualise a person's DNA as an instruction manual for constructing and operating that particular person.

Like any other book, a manual is composed of sentences and words written in a language – Welsh, Urdu, English and so on – which has meaning to anyone who understands the rules of that language. So a language is a form of code. In the kind of language that you and I understand, the meaning is conveyed by letters of the alphabet, their sequence and the way that they are grouped together.

The DNA manual is also 'written' in a language or code – the genetic code. It exists in the actual structure of DNA, which we could think of as a 'living book'. The 'letters' in which it is written are the sub-units from which the DNA is built up and the meaning is conveyed by the sequence of these sub-units and the way that they are grouped together.

The English alphabet contains 26 letters. Other languages have more or less, but always an appreciable number. There are only four different sub-units in DNA and so the DNA language has only four 'letters'. All DNA is composed of long chains of these sub-units. They are usually identified by the initial letters of their chemical names – A, T, C and G. So a section of DNA chain could be shown as a series of these four letters, indicating the order of the sub-units in that part of the chain. For example … ATTGGCTAGT … and so on.

This series of letters spells out a section of the genetic code. Although we ourselves cannot read it, it has meaning inside the living cell. In order to make this meaning clear, I am going to draw on some material from the biochemistry unit.

All living cells carry out complex activities which make up the actual process of living. These activities are brought about by **proteins** – which can be thought of as the cell's machinery. The kind of work that any particular cell can do depends on the proteins which it produces at any given time. So it should be clear that proteins are the key to the cell's activities, and ultimately to the well-being of the whole body. Thus the genetic information carried in the nucleus has to control this most fundamental of processes, the manufacture of proteins.

This is exactly what the DNA code does. All proteins are built up from small building blocks called **amino acids**. The nature of a protein depends on the order in which the amino acids are joined together, and the DNA code spells out the order in which this is to happen when a protein is made.

Just as the letters in an instruction book are grouped together to form words, so the DNA sub-units are grouped to form units of meaning which we can think of as 'words'. Unlike the book, all the DNA words are the same length. They are all three letters – or three sub-units – long. For that reason, they are termed **triplets** and the DNA code is known as a **triplet code**.

Figure 5 shows the relationship between the DNA words and the proteins which are made in the cell.

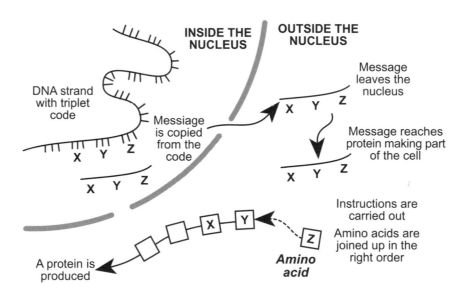

Figure 5 The relationship between DNA and protein manufacture

Inside the nucleus the DNA message is copied onto **RNA** - the second type of nucleic acid. RNA is very similar to DNA , but it exists in smaller fragments which can easily pass out of the nucleus (through pores in the nuclear membrane) and so transmit the message written in the DNA. The way in which the code is copied is described in section 4.1 and the synthesis of proteins is detailed in the biochemistry unit of this series.

The parts of the cell which manufacture proteins recognise triplet words. Each word specifies where a particular amino acid should go when the cellular machinery is making a protein. Each one means: 'Put this amino acid here when you make a protein.'

The piece of code shown in *Figure 5* contains three words, reading from left to right: att/ggc/tag/t, and so on. Each word specifies a different amino acid. So suppose that:

ATT   =   amino acid 'X'
GGC   =   amino acid 'Y'
TAG   =   amino acid 'Z

then this piece of code will instruct the cell to make a protein in which x, y and z are joined together in that order.

In the next activity, I want you to write a piece of genetic code for yourself, and begin to think about the effect of making a mistake.

ACTIVITY 8 — ALLOW 5 MINUTES

The DNA code word for amino acid B is ATA.

1 Write a piece of code which will instruct the cell to join three Bs together.

2 Then write it out again, but this time make a deliberate mistake with the fourth letter along from the left. You could miss it out, put it in twice, or change it for another letter.

3 Now look at your piece of code and see what the effect will be on the instructions which it gives to the cell.

Commentary

The piece of code you're looking for is:

... ATA ATA ATA ...

Your answer to the first part of the activity depends on the principle that the genetic code is based on groups of three letters, always read in the same direction, which I have shown as left to right.

This principle is not always easy to follow the first time, because it requires us to deal with abstractions. So if you didn't get the answer right this time, don't worry – you're certainly not alone! Try reading through 'The genetic code' again, and follow the argument step by step.

Here are some of the things you might have done for the second part of the activity:

- delete a letter   ATA TA ATA
- add a letter   ATAA ATA ATA
- replace a letter   ATA GTA ATA

In each of these cases, you will find that – reading from left to right in groups of three – you get a different set of 'words'.

Deleting a letter gives   ATA TAA TA?

This gives one amino acid B, followed by two different amino acids.

Addition gives you   ATA AAT AAT A??

Again, the first amino acid in the protein chain is amino acid B, but the others will be different.

Replacing a letter gives   ATA GTA ATA

The first and third amino acids are B, but the middle one is different.

The result of all three kinds of mistake is a piece of code which is different from the original sequence. If this happens to the code for part of a protein, the resulting protein will obviously be slightly different from the original.

Variation in the code

What you have just done is a pencil and paper exercise which mirrors what can and does happen in the cell. It shows how a change in the code changes the order of the amino acids from which the proteins are made up.

But does this matter?

In the next activity, we'll look at an example of the effects of a change in the code, and the resultant change in some very important proteins.

ACTIVITY 9   ALLOW 15 MINUTES

Please read through the following case study, and then note your answers to the questions that follow it.

Karima is a very ill eight-month-old baby. She was born in London to parents who arrived there from Pakistan three years ago.

She was a healthy baby, delivered normally, and was well for the first three months of her life. She began to show a failure to thrive, and has now been admitted to a children's ward with profound anaemia. She has recurrent fevers and an enlarged spleen, causing her abdomen to be very distended.

Her parents are very worried because Karima had a little brother who died at the age of three, after showing similar symptoms a few months after he was born. As time went on, he failed to grow and his legs became deformed.

Karima's parents have two other children, both well. Her mother has just found that she is pregnant again, and both parents had younger sisters who died in infancy of a severe type of anaemia.

Karima is diagnosed as having a type of blood disorder called thalassaemia, and is given immediate treatment for the anaemia. Her mother is offered a test to check the DNA of the new baby before it is born.

1 Now that you have read about Karima's illness – thalassaemia – identify the systems of the body which it affects.

2 Do you think that this illness is caused by genetic or environmental factors, or by a combination of the two?

Commentary

Your answers should have been along the following lines.

1 The illness affected Karima's blood system, giving rise to the anaemia and the enlarged spleen. In her brother's case, it affected his skeleton too, since his limbs were deformed. As her brother died, there must also have been far-reaching effects on other body systems.

2 At first sight, it seems as if this condition is due to genetic factors. It runs in this family, and the mother is offered a genetic test on the unborn baby. However, the fact that the illness started several months after birth is a bit puzzling. Is this really a genetic effect or could environmental factors have been involved? It is difficult to say without further information.

A fuller explanation of Karima's case

Thalassaemia is an inherited illness. It results in a failure to make the oxygen carrying part of the blood, **haemoglobin (Hb)**, properly. This results in anaemia.

The unborn child has a type of haemoglobin (**foetal Hb**) which is slightly different from the adult type (**adult Hb**). It picks up oxygen more easily, and so can extract oxygen from the mother's blood as it flows through the placenta. When the baby is born, it continues to use foetal Hb for a few months, but soon needs to start making adult Hb. This is when the trouble starts for a child with thalassaemia.

The problem is that part of the genetic code responsible for the production of adult Hb contains a mistake in people who suffer from this illness. The part responsible for foetal Hb is not affected. The baby is well at first, but cannot make adult Hb when the time comes. The child therefore becomes more and more anaemic.

In an attempt to increase the output of this vital protein, the blood-forming tissues of the body increase in volume. Thus the spleen and bone marrow (the place where red-blood cells are made) get larger, causing the abdomen to swell and bones to become distorted. Without treatment, this form of the disease leads to severe illness and death.

As you read the description of the severity of these symptoms, you may have wondered about the nature of the genetic 'mistake' which could have such far-reaching effects. This is known to be due to a single mistake, like the one you made in *Activity 8*. It is actually due to a replacement in the code, which changes a single amino acid in part of the adult Hb molecule. Because this oxygen-carrying substance is so central to all the activities of living, this apparently insignificant change has very widespread consequences.

I provided this example to demonstrate what a small change in a crucial part of the genetic code can do. It produces a malfunction, and therefore constitutes a mistake in the code.

However, there are many ways in which the code can vary without producing adverse effects – just slight differences of the kind that we have been observing in healthy people.

Within each nucleus there is a great deal of DNA. It is calculated that, if all the DNA in a nucleus were to be unravelled and stretched out, it would be approximately two metres in length and would contain something like three billion (3,000,000,000) sub-units.

There are so many possible places for the code to vary that each person has a unique genetic code – their **DNA fingerprint**. No two people, apart from identical twins, have exactly the same sequence of units in their DNA. Nowadays, it is possible for geneticists to work out the sequence in the nuclei of living or dead cells. This is why small samples of hair or skin can be used to track down criminals. The sequence of the DNA code found in their cells can be matched against those of people suspected of the crime.

Here we have an explanation of the source of the genetic diversity of the human race. Each person starts life with a unique set of genetic code in the fertilised egg. This leads us to ask more questions, such as how do the differences in the code arise? We'll consider this subject in the next section, but first here is a summary of the main points covered in this section.

Summary of Section 5

- The nuclei of all cells contain DNA.

- DNA carries genetic information in the form of the genetic code.

- This information determines the manufacture of proteins.

- The code is written in the sequence of DNA sub-units (A, T, G and C).

- Code 'words' are groups of three sub-units called triplets.

- Each triplet word specifies the position of an amino acid in a protein.

- Small changes in the code are responsible for variation.

- Some changes cause malfunctions.

- Each person has a unique genetic sequence.

6: Mixing the code

As you know, the fertilised egg is all that we have to start life with, and all of our instruction manual is contained in it. So now let's see how each person comes to have a unique set of instructions.

ACTIVITY 10   ALLOW 5 MINUTES

Read the following two paragraphs, and then note down your answers to the questions that follow.

The fertilised egg is formed at conception by the union of an egg and a sperm. The sperm is formed in the father's testes. It is sometimes described as a 'naked nucleus', because it contains very little besides the nucleus and a tail which allows it to move actively. The egg is larger because it contains a nucleus and all the other components of a cell, and also a food store to start the growth of the embryo. It is formed in the mother's ovary.

At fertilisation, many sperm cluster on the outside of the egg but only one succeeds in penetrating its outer layer. The sperm nucleus is propelled into the egg and fuses with the egg nucleus to make the single nucleus of the fertilised egg, which then starts to divide and eventually forms the embryo.

1   What does the sperm donate to the fertilised egg?

2   What does the nucleus of the fertilised egg contain?

3   Your parents both contributed genetic material to the fertilised egg from which you grew. In turn, your four grandparents contributed genetic material to your parents and hence to you. Can you work out how many people in total have handed down some of their genetic material to you in the past hundred years? You may find it helpful to set this out as a diagram, starting with yourself and working back to your great-great grandparents.

Commentary

The answers are as follows:

1 The sperm contributes only its nucleus. That is all it contains, and therefore the DNA in the nucleus is all that the male parent can give to the fertilised egg.

2 The fertilised egg contains the contents of the egg nucleus and the sperm nucleus. In other words, it contains both maternal and paternal DNA.

These first two questions should have reinforced the idea that all the information passed from generation to generation is found in the egg at conception.

3 You had 16 great-great-grandparents, so the instruction book in your fertilised egg contains contributions from all of them. In other words, your DNA is a mixture made up from all of theirs. *Figure 6* shows how this comes about.

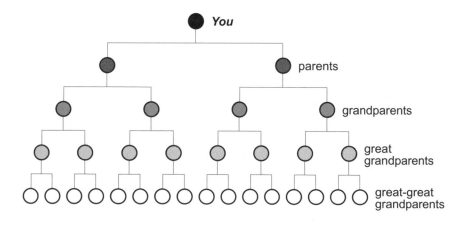

Figure 6 Contributors to your genetic mixture

The human race has been on earth for thousands of years, so over that time your DNA has had contributions from literally millions of your ancestors. Your own set of ancestors is different from everyone else's, except your brothers and sisters, so your DNA is a unique mixture. That is what makes you different from anyone else.

But, you may say, 'What about my brothers and sisters? I'm not like them', or 'If I had any, I know I would not be the same unless we were identical twins'.

Of course, you are quite right. Even though you and your siblings share the same set of ancestors, you do not have the same set of genes unless you are twins who grew from the same fertilised egg. This is because when sexual reproduction takes place a mixing process occurs which results in each child getting a different mix from the same set of parental genes. It is rather like the process of shuffling and dealing several hands from the same pack of cards, and is a major source of additional variation.

Before you can appreciate this process fully, you need more information about the packaging and distribution of genetic material. This is the subject of the next section.

7: Organising the code

Many people associate the science of genetics with genes and chromosomes. You may have been wondering when this topic would be covered. I felt it was important to provide you with an understanding of the nature of the genetic code first, so that you could form a picture of the material from which genes and chromosomes are made and therefore understand how they function. So now we will take a look at the way that the DNA is organised.

The human genome

In describing the genetic code, I used the metaphor of an instruction manual and described the units of meaning – or words – from which it is written. Let's take the metaphor a stage further now and think about the sentences in the manual.

In ordinary language, a sentence is a set of words dealing with one topic. In DNA code, the words are arranged in sequences, each one dealing with a single activity, so we could call them sentences, too. A gene is such a sentence. It is a section of the nuclear DNA containing many triplet 'words'. It deals with either of the following topics:

- making a specific protein

- controlling the activities of other genes.

Genes with related functions are known to be grouped together. For example, several genes in a cluster are involved in the production of the protein chains of the various forms of haemoglobin. In Karima's case study, I explained that the baby switches from foetal to adult Hb early in life. There is one gene to control the production of each of these proteins. As the baby grows, the foetal Hb gene is switched off and the adult Hb gene is switched on. This is done by a **regulator gene** which lies close to them.

Regulator genes are of great importance in maintaining the correct sequence of growth and development in the cell. When they go wrong, the consequence may be uncontrolled growth, which we will consider in Session Four of this unit.

Since each gene is a section of the nuclear DNA, it is subject to the variation which we have already considered. The 'sentence' can be spelled in a number of different ways and still make sense. Many normal genes, therefore, exist in two or more alternative forms. These alternatives result in slight differences in the proteins which they produce.

However, if a sentence contains too many spelling mistakes in important places it will cease to make sense, or will make the wrong kind of sense. For example, the sentence, 'Show these ladies into their seats' will have the desired effect. But 'Sew these ladies into their sheets' will cause some confusion, even though it is still a meaningful sentence.

In the same way, some changes in the code produce genes which function incorrectly or fail to function entirely. When discussing Karima's illness, I told you that there was a small mistake in part of the DNA. One of the triplet 'words' was wrongly spelt. Perhaps you can see that the result of this is an incorrect 'sentence' – in other words, a faulty gene.

Mapping the human genome

The complete set of genes which humans possess is called the **human genome**. There are believed to be about 100,000 genes in the human genome.

At present, scientists throughout the world are working on a collaborative project to make a complete map of the genome. In the course of this work, the structure of several genes has been worked out. Once this has been done, the gene can be produced in the laboratory. This then opens up the possibility of replacing a faulty gene in an affected person's cells with a good copy.

In theory, a good adult Hb gene could be made and used to treat Karima. The problem is, how could such a gene be inserted correctly into Karima's DNA?

ACTIVITY 11　　　ALLOW 5 MINUTES

First, read the short report of the paper on gene therapy for muscular dystrophy (*Resource 2*). This is provided as an example of the possibilities that are opening up in the field of gene replacement.

As you read it, note down how the author suggests that the dystrophin gene could be inserted into cells.

Commentary

The paper suggests that the gene could be inserted by the use of a **retrovirus**. You may not have met this term before. It refers to a particular type of virus which can carry genes into human cells. Before explaining this further, I would like to discuss briefly the nature of viruses to show how they could be used in **gene therapy** – that is, the replacement of faulty genes.

Viruses

Most people identify viruses as the cause of a number of minor illnesses, such as colds and flu. It seems that a convenient diagnosis for unexplained minor illnesses is, 'It's just a virus that's going about'.

Viruses are very commonplace, but they are also very unusual. The next activity demonstrates one of their unusual features.

ACTIVITY 12   ALLOW 5 MINUTES

Think about the last time you had a really bad cold or a bout of flu, or about anyone in your family who has recently had a viral illness such as mumps, measles, chicken-pox or shingles.

1   What treatment is usually advised for a bad cold or for flu?

2   Does the treatment include antibiotic therapy?

3   Are antibiotics given to people who are suffering from mumps or measles?

4   What reasons can you give for your answers to the second and third questions?

Commentary

Usually the treatment advised for colds and flu is rest, fluids and mild analgesia. Antibiotics are not given unless there is a bacterial infection in addition to the viral one. The same is true for the other viral illnesses.

This is because antibiotics have no effect on viruses. Antibiotics kill bacteria by interfering with the processes which go on inside their living cells. Viruses do not have cellular structures and processes. They consist of nucleic acids inside a protein shell whose function it is to get the virus into the nucleus of a living cell. Once inside, the virus takes over the genetic code of that cell – the **host** cell – and alters the host genes in such a way that they make new virus particles.

Some viruses do a lot of damage to the host in this process. Others are relatively benign and go undetected or cause only a minor ailment, such as a cold sore. Their ability to get into cells presents a possible means of introducing 'good' genes into the cells of people who are ill as a result of having faulty genes. If the good genes can be manufactured and spliced into the viral nucleic acid, they could be taken into the nuclei of the affected cells. This is the basis of the optimism about the possibilities for gene therapy.

Retroviruses are particularly useful because they consist of RNA rather than DNA, and have the unique ability to make DNA from it. With suitable techniques, these viruses can be 'tailored' to induce the cells they enter to make good copies of the pieces of DNA which are faulty. So they can induce the cells of an affected person to manufacture their own good genes.

This unique ability of the retrovirus is possible because these viruses depend on chemical processes which are not found in any other plant or animal cells. It is also their vulnerable point. If a drug could be found to block these processes, it would be active against the virus but would not affect the human cells infected by the virus. The search for this kind of drug is intense at present because the **Human immunodeficiency virus (HIV)** is a retrovirus. Drug therapy for the serious conditions which result from HIV infection may therefore depend on this approach.

Since viruses are essentially pieces of nucleic acid that can only function inside living cell nuclei, they are considered by some geneticists to be 'escaped genes'.

One theory goes that they are very successful because they can hijack the nuclei of living cells and get them to do their work for them. Those viruses which have been associated with the human species for a very long time usually do little harm to their human hosts. It is in the best interest of the virus not to kill off its host species. Therefore viruses have gradually come to be less damaging to their hosts by the process of natural selection, which we will consider in Session Three. The host also becomes more tolerant of the virus; the overall result is that host and virus are adapted to one another and the virus does very little harm to the host.

However, viruses which have recently invaded a species tend to be very damaging. This is certainly the case with those which have just entered the human species, such as HIV.

In theory, harmless viruses could be used to carry good genes into defective cells. The problem is that there is a limited understanding of what else an altered virus might do if it was liberated from the defective cells, found its way into other parts of the body or was passed from person to person. Gene therapy will only become viable when these problems have been tackled and overcome.

We are going to hear a lot more about the problems and possibilities of gene therapy in the immediate future, and I hope that this brief introduction will help you to feel better informed about this important subject. There are some references to up-to-date works on this topic in the Further Reading section at the end of this unit.

At this point you will probably find it useful to have a brief summary of the previous two sections.

Summary of Sections 6 and 7

- The nucleus of the fertilised egg contains a mixture of maternal and paternal DNA.

- A gene is a section of the nuclear DNA dealing with the control of a single cellular activity.

- The activity may be the production of a protein or the regulation of other genes.

- Genes can exist in alternative forms.

- Some changes in genes lead to faulty genes which are malfunctional.

- Genes with related activities tend to be grouped together.

- The complete set of human genes is the genome.

- Faulty genes could be replaced through gene therapy if a way could be found to insert them into the cells of affected people.

- Viruses are pieces of nucleic acid with the ability to insert themselves into living cell nuclei.

- Harmless viruses could be a vehicle for gene therapy.

Now we can move on from the study of genes to the next level of organisation of the genetic material – the chromosomes.

8: Human chromosomes

Up to this point, I have used the metaphor of a book to help you visualise the nature of the genetic code. Here is a short activity to review the terms that have been used, and to lead on to a consideration of the function of chromosomes.

ACTIVITY 13   ALLOW 5 MINUTES

Below you will find two lists of words. The list on the left is of words which have been used in the previous sections. The list on the right contains words we use in talking about the sorts of material we find in books. See if you can pair the words correctly by connecting them with arrows.

A) DNA   1) letters
B) triplets   2) book
C) groups of genes   3) sentences
D) genes   4) words
E) sub-units   5) paragraphs

Commentary

According to the metaphor that we've been using, the correct pairings are as follows:

E and 1:   sub-units and letters
B and 4:   triplets and words
D and 3:   genes and sentences
C and 5:   groups of genes and paragraphs
A and 2:   DNA and the book

I have not yet used a metaphor for the chromosomes, but since they come between the paragraph and the whole book, it would be reasonable to refer to them as chapters.

Each chromosome is composed of many groups of genes. They are the structures in which the genes are organised at the time of cell division. *Figure 7* shows in diagrammatic form the nucleus of a dividing cell in the skin.

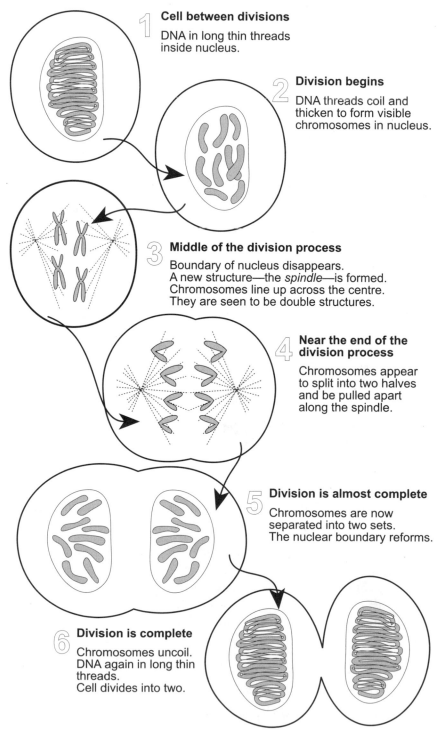

1 Cell between divisions

DNA in long thin threads inside nucleus.

2 Division begins

DNA threads coil and thicken to form visible chromosomes in nucleus.

3 Middle of the division process

Boundary of nucleus disappears. A new structure—the *spindle*—is formed. Chromosomes line up across the centre. They are seen to be double structures.

4 Near the end of the division process

Chromosomes appear to split into two halves and be pulled apart along the spindle.

5 Division is almost complete

Chromosomes are now separated into two sets. The nuclear boundary reforms.

6 Division is complete

Chromosomes uncoil. DNA again in long thin threads. Cell divides into two.

Figure 7 A dividing cell

Figure 7 emphasises what happens to the DNA and the chromosomes. This is not a complete picture of the mechanics of cell division, and I have not included details of all the structures involved or the names of the various phases. I want you to concentrate on what the DNA does when cells divide.

The type of division shown here is **mitosis**, the type that occurs in all cells of the body except the sex cells. When eggs and sperm are produced a more complex form of cell division is needed – **meiosis** – which will be described in Session Two.

In *Figure 7*, you can see that the chromosomes appear as the nucleus starts to divide. It is worth stressing this point, because people are sometimes puzzled as to what the chromosomes are for. Having seen photographs of the chromosomes in the dividing nucleus, some people assume that these bodies actually represent the internal structure of the nucleus. In fact, they are only seen at this time and they represent a way of 'packaging' the DNA so that it can be equally divided between the daughters. Once cell division is complete, the chromosomes are 'unpacked' to allow the DNA to resume its functions.

Let's consider this in a little more detail. When the cell is not actively dividing, the genes in the long DNA threads are active in controlling the manufacture of proteins and thus the activities of the cell. No distinct structure can be seen. This is sometimes called the **resting nucleus** – a rather misleading name as the nucleus is actually very active at this time.

When the cell is about to divide, it has to do two things:

- The DNA must be copied so that there are two complete 'sets', one for each daughter cell

- The DNA must be organised in some way so that it can be equally shared out to the 'daughter' cells.

Just before any changes are visible in a nucleus which has started to divide, chemical tests show that it contains twice as much DNA as before. In response to some signal telling the cell that it is time to divide, the DNA is copied – the correct term is 'replicated'. Once this has happened, the DNA threads begin a process of coiling and shortening, which makes them many times thicker than they were, so they become visible under the microscope. It is at this point that the structures we call chromosomes become recognisable.

Because there are now two batches of DNA in the nucleus, each chromosome is a double structure. The two halves of each one are the same, with the same genes in the same sequence. The two halves are joined at one or more points along their length. The length and position of the joining point are characteristic of each chromosome and enable them to be identified.

Dividing nuclei can be stained and squashed so that the chromosomes are spread out and easy to see and photograph. The photographic image can be cut up and the chromosomes arranged in rows, as shown in *Figure 8*.

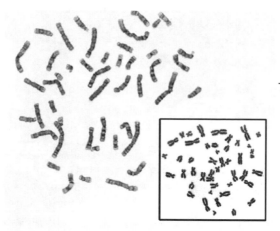

Figure 8a

Nucleus squashed to show separate chromosomes

The 46 chromosomes from a single male cell undergoing mitosis(inset),and from the same blood culture a mitotic cell treated in the laboratory with a short exposure to enzyme trypsin then stained to reveal linear bands along the chromosome.

Figure 8b

This is actually Figure 8a cut up and rearranged to show paired chromosomes

The same 46 doubled chromosomes as in Figure 8a. They are arranged in decreasing order of size and numbered from 1 to 22. The sex chromosomes are shown as X and Y. The letters A to G show the groups of chromosomes. Individual pairs of chromosomes in any of the groups can now be identified by banding patterns.

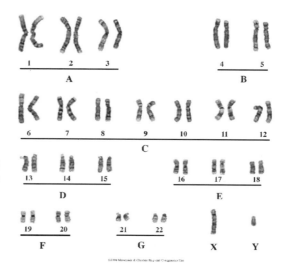

Figure 8 Human chromosomes

If you study this display, you will see that the chromosomes are grouped in similar pairs, each pair except one being identical in length and shape. I will explain the reason for this in Session Two.

The next activity provides an opportunity for you to revise your understanding of this process and to see what happens next.

ACTIVITY 14 — ALLOW 10 MINUTES

Study the diagrams of a dividing nucleus, shown overleaf as *Figure 9*. Then fill in the blank spaces in the text alongside the drawings of each stage in the process.

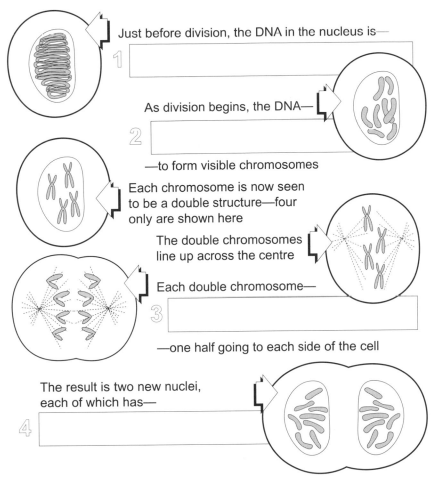

Just before division, the DNA in the nucleus is—

1

As division begins, the DNA—

2

—to form visible chromosomes

Each chromosome is now seen to be a double structure—four only are shown here

The double chromosomes line up across the centre

Each double chromosome—

3

—one half going to each side of the cell

The result is two new nuclei, each of which has—

4

Figure 9

Commentary

1 You may have written down 'doubled', 'copied' or 'replicated' – in fact, any word which indicates that a copy is made of the DNA and therefore of all the genes.

2 You needed to convey the idea that the long DNA threads become shorter and thicker, forming the chromosomes which can now be seen. Words like 'coils', 'condenses' and 'wound up' are appropriate here.

3 This diagram shows that each double chromosome 'splits' or 'divides', one half going to each end of the nucleus.

4 You should have written something along the lines of, 'The same number of single chromosomes as the parent cell'.

This diagram should help you to envisage what happens during mitosis, the type of division which occurs in growing tissues, healing wounds and in the developing embryo. Here is a summary of the key points about DNA and mitosis.

Summary of Section 8

● Mitosis is the cell division which occurs during growth and repair.

● At the start of mitosis, DNA is replicated.

- The DNA then coils up to form the chromosomes.

- Each chromosome is a double structure at this stage.

- Each double chromosome carries two copies of each gene.

- When the nucleus divides, the double chromosomes split apart, so that each new nucleus has the same number and type of genes as the parent.

This explanation of what happens to the chromosomes when cells divide leaves us with a rather awkward question. You may be saying to yourself, 'If all the cells contain the same DNA as their parents, why are they not all the same? Why and how do the cells of the embryo turn into the different parts of the growing baby?' These are very important questions, and we will consider them in the next section.

9: Why the difference?

In any kind of healing wound – whether surgical, traumatic or chronic – cell division is occurring. If the function of the affected area is to be restored, it is vital for the injured tissues to resume their original structure.

By studying the process of wound healing, we can gain an insight into the factors which influence the development of cells after they have divided.

ACTIVITY 15   ALLOW **20** MINUTES

Please read the *Resource 3*, on wound healing, in the Resource Section. As you do so, make a list of the factors which affect wound healing. In other words, indicate those factors that influence the cells which have divided to develop in a particular way.

Commentary

I'm sure that you will have identified some of the following factors:

- the temperature of the wound
- the degree of humidity at the healing surface
- the oxygen tension in the wound
- the patient's nutritional status
- the presence of foreign material in the wound
- the spatial relationship of the healing surfaces
  – along with many other similar factors.

All of these factors relate to the *environment* in which the cells are dividing. The cells may have the potential to divide and to develop into healed tissue, but this can only be achieved if the external surroundings are right.

The environment affects the way that the genes in a particular cell work out – that is, the way in which they are *expressed*. If the environment in the healing wound is wrong, the cells will turn into scar tissue rather than the appropriate skin and connective tissues.

The same is true of the developing embryo. The process by which cells that are genetically the same turn into all the different tissues in the baby is termed **differentiation**, and it is not fully understood by scientists at present. However, the environment and the position of the cells in the very early embryo are known to affect the way in which they develop.

We can apply the same principle to the whole person, too, since the way that the genes in the cells are expressed determines all the inherited characteristics of the person. Each human being has a unique genetic potential, governed by their individual set of DNA. The extent to which that potential is achieved depends upon the person's physical and social environment.

When the person is a patient or client receiving health care, the health practitioner is a vital element of the environment and can assist the person to achieve their potential under the particular circumstances.

For example, the health visitor has a vital role with children under five years old in detecting sensory impairment – such as deafness – at an early stage. A child may have considerable intellectual potential, but early undetected deafness caused by repeated ear infections can interfere with speech acquisition and result in a slow start at school. The health visitor is concerned to minimise the adverse effects of the environment on the development of the child's genetic potential.

So we see that, in all levels of life, from the cell to the whole person, the forces of genetics and the environment interact. So let's finish off this first section by applying this principle to the study of some real people.

10: Looking at patients and clients

At the beginning of this unit, I asked you to observe the variation which exists between groups of people. We can do this for the people in our care, too. By becoming aware of the variation between people with the same health problem, we become more aware of the meaning of 'individualised patient care'.

ACTIVITY 16   ALLOW **30** MINUTES

Here are two short case studies of women who are the patients of the same GP, and are under the care of the same consultant oncologist. These studies are based on real people, although their names and other details have been changed, for obvious reasons. Both women have a diagnosis of carcinoma of the breast. Please read through the case studies, and then follow the instructions at the end.

Mary

Mary is now 36 and married with two young children – a son aged five and a daughter aged 18 months. Her cancer was diagnosed when she was pregnant with her second child. She noticed a breast lump right at the start of her pregnancy, but was told that it was nothing to worry about. Later, she sought a second opinion and the lump was found to be malignant.

She has had the breast and some tissue under her arm removed. The skin at the operation site has formed a large mass of scar tissue which stands out from the front wall of her chest.

Mary was well for a year after the operation and pursued an active policy of self-help, visiting various centres and finding out about alternative therapies. She put herself on a very strict diet of fresh fruit and vegetables, and was considering further surgery to remove the scar tissue.

Unfortunately, three months ago she began to suffer from pain and nausea. Investigations showed that she has secondary cancers in her liver and in some bones. Mary's mother died from breast cancer before she was 40. Mary is very aware that her outlook is poor, but she is amazingly calm and positive – on the outside, at least. She leads an active life with her husband and children when she feels well enough to do so.

Pauline

Pauline also has breast cancer. She is 82, a widow living alone. Two of her sons live nearby and she has a supportive family, including two great-grandchildren of whom she is especially fond.

Her cancer was only discovered when she came into Casualty recently after fracturing her wrist in a fall one winter morning. The fracture was treated under general anaesthetic, and when the staff removed her clothing they found that she had a large, ulcerating mass where her left breast should have been. Obviously she had concealed this for a number of years.

Apart from the ulcer itself, Pauline is reasonably well for her age. She is able to get about and enjoys the company of her family and friends. There is no evident sign that the cancer has spread to other parts of her body.

Pauline seems to totally disregard the ulcer. She doesn't like to talk about it much, and reckons that 'It's just part of getting old'. To the best of her knowledge, none of her close female relatives have had breast cancer.

Now that you have read the case studies, make a list of the differences which can be observed between these two women. For each one that you identify, decide on its major source. Is it genetic, environmental, or a combination of the two?

You'll find it helpful to read *Resource 4* when you are analysing these differences. It is very readable, and it contains up-to-date information about the part that inheritance plays in some types of breast cancer, as well as details of other inherited health tendencies.

Commentary

There are at least five differences between these two women in relation to their illness.

1. The time of onset. Mary was 34 when her cancer was diagnosed; Pauline was 82.

2. The rate of progress of the disease. Mary had a very rapid onset and soon developed bone and liver secondary cancers. Pauline had her cancer for a long time before anyone else knew about it – possibly several years.

3. The manifestation of the disease. Mary had surgery to remove the entire breast. She has extensive scar formation at the site. Pauline concealed her condition and has not had any surgery. She now has a large ulcerating mass at the site, but no evidence of further spread.

4. Their family histories. Pauline cannot recall any relative with the same illness. However, Mary's mother died of breast cancer at an early age.

5. The method of coping. Mary is very active and energetic, and is using every method she can, including alternative therapies, to combat the disease. She maintains an optimistic outlook for the sake of her young family. Pauline considers that this is all part of growing old and has effectively ignored the slowly developing ulcer for many years.

Sources of variation

The sources of variation could be described in the following terms:

1. The time of onset could well be genetically determined. From *Resource 4*, you will see that there appears to be a genetic cause for some early-onset breast cancer. However, environmental factors such as Mary's pregnancy could also play a part.

2. Mary's cancer started early and grew when her body was undergoing the hormonal changes of pregnancy. So the cancer cells grew in an internal environment where levels of hormones were fluctuating. Hormones affect cellular growth. It is therefore likely that this environment will have influenced the rate of growth of Mary's cancer. It could also be that genetic factors produced two different types of cancer in these two women.

3. Much of the difference between the manifestation of these two cancers is due to environmental factors. Mary has had surgery and Pauline has not.

4. In Mary's case, the family history shows a genetic basis for the observed difference.

5. The different methods of coping adopted by each woman depend on both genetic and environmental factors. Each woman has certain inborn characteristics which have been shaped by her life experiences to produce the strengths which she is showing at this time.

You will see that for nearly all these differences, a mixture of genetic and environmental causes can be demonstrated. The combined action of these causes results in two people who have the same medical diagnosis but very different needs.

When planning care for two such people, these differences and their underlying causes need to be taken into account. They help us to understand the reasons for a person's present situation and their reactions to it. This understanding is necessary so that we can make the most appropriate and helpful response. By gaining a clearer view of the potential of each patient or client we can work with them to identify realistic goals and to assess progress towards meeting these. Finally, our understanding of genetic variation provides us with a way of looking at the important people in the lives of our patients and clients, since these people are part of the environment and many of them are linked genetically to the person receiving care.

Summary of Sections 9 and 10

- The way in which genes are expressed depends on environmental factors.

- This applies at the levels both of the cell and of the whole person.

- Observed variation in patients and clients is due to a combination of genetic and environmental factors.

You have now reached the end of Session One. Before you move on to Session Two, check that you have achieved the objectives given at the beginning of this session, and, if not, review the appropriate sections.

SESSION TWO

Randomness

Introduction

The second idea that I would like to explore in this unit is that of randomness; that is to say, the occurrence of random events. This will lead us to a discussion of how certain mathematical predictions about inheritance can be made. Some people are put off the study of genetics by its numerical aspects. I hope to show you here that it is possible to study important and interesting parts of the subject without the need for any mathematics at all.

In this section, we will explore what random events are, and then use this understanding to describe the way that sex is determined and how mistakes in the genetic code can occur.

We will then think about characteristics which show clear-cut patterns of inheritance, and those in which the situation is more complex because many genes are involved.

This will lead on to the idea of continuous variation, its causes and the way it leads us to the establishment of the human characteristics we have come to think of as normal.

Session objectives

When you have completed this session you should be able to:

- explain the random nature of the inheritance of gender
- explain how an understanding of the role of randomness in cell division enables genetic outcomes to be predicted
- outline the basis of single-factor inheritance patterns
- explain how random events contribute to genetic variation
- describe the contribution of genes and the environment to the establishment of a 'normal' state
- apply the ideas in this session to care planning.

Please note this text is written so that it can be understood by people who have not studied genetics at all in the past. It may be you have already achieved these outcomes and wish to use the material for revision purposes.

1: The nature of random events

The ability of genetic science to make predictions about inheritance patterns depends on the random nature of genetic events. The following activity will help you to appreciate what random events are. We will then apply this understanding to the events which take place during cell division and fertilisation.

ACTIVITY 17   ALLOW **30** MINUTES

For this activity I would like you to try a simple experiment that involves tossing a coin. Before you begin, jot down your answer to the following question:

'Each time a coin is tossed, what is the chance that it will come down "heads"?'

Now toss the coin one hundred times. Each time, record its fall as 'H' or 'T' (heads or tails). Add up the number of each, and record your result.

Commentary

Your answer to the question was probably 50/50, or something similar – 'half and half', 'one chance in two', or 'evens'. This was probably something you knew by instinct.

The coin-tossing experiment showed whether you were correct. You would expect to find that the coin fell 'heads' on about half of the tosses. So when this experiment is performed, the outcome will often be close to fifty heads and fifty tails.

However, you may have found something quite different. It is perfectly possible – although extremely unlikely – that you got 100 heads or 100 tails. But if you added your score to that of all the other people who have done this experiment, the overall score would inevitably approach equal numbers of heads and tails.

This is because tossing a coin is a random event. The outcome of this event – the way the coin falls – is due to many different factors which don't show any particular pattern. There is no one major influence on the way the coin falls.

However, if the coin is bent or weighted in some way, this will strongly influence the way it falls. There will then be a predictable pattern, and therefore tossing this coin will not be a random event.

When things occur randomly – with no clear pattern and no main cause – we usually say that the outcome is 'due to chance alone'.

Check your understanding of this in the next activity.

ACTIVITY 18   ALLOW **5** MINUTES

Consider the events in the list below. Tick each one which you think is a random event, where the outcome is due to chance alone.

1 Taking an exam ☐
2 Having a baby ☐
3 Dealing a hand at cards ☐

4   Queuing at the checkout   ☐
5   Giving an injection   ☐

Commentary

I guess that you rapidly concluded that number three is a random event (assuming that no one is cheating) and that the length of time you wait at the checkout is also due to chance.

When taking an exam, the outcome should not be the result of chance alone.

But what about the other two? They don't sound like random events, but in some senses they are. This depends on the outcome on which we choose to focus.

In giving an injection, if the outcome studied was 'bruising', then there is an element of chance about whether this occurs or not. It depends on whether the needle hits a small blood vessel or not. So giving an injection is a random event in relation to bruising.

The birth of a baby is a random event in terms of the outcome, 'sex of the baby' unless, as sometimes occurs, some intervention has taken place to ensure that a foetus of one sex does not come to term.

We will be using estimates of chance for random events like this in the following section, so we need to express them in a form which everyone can use. When we say, 'fifty/fifty', this is the same thing as saying 'one chance in two'. In genetics, this is expressed as a fraction. So 'one chance in two' becomes 'one over two', or '½'.

ACTIVITY 19   ALLOW 3 MINUTES

If the idea of expressing chance in this way is new to you, here is an activity to help.

Suggest a fraction in answer to the following question:
'When you throw a dice, what is the chance that you'll get a six?'

Commentary

Common sense tells us that, since the dice can fall six different ways there is a one in six chance of getting any particular score. So the chance of getting a six is one chance in six, or one over six, or ⅙.

You can arrive at an answer like this because you have knowledge of the way in which the world works. We live in a world full of random events, and although you may not have been aware of the fact, you do understand the nature of random events.

This understanding is the basis of probability theory, which underlies mathematical genetics. However, this is not some abstract concept with no practical use. We apply it in everyday life more than we might realise. Unconsciously, we weigh up the costs and benefits of any particular action and we base this on our instinctive knowledge about the probability that certain things will – or will not – happen. This is also true in health care, as the following activity illustrates.

ACTIVITY 20

ALLOW 5 MINUTES

Imagine that you are working in primary health care and a mother visits you. She is worried about having her child immunised against a certain disease before travelling abroad. You look up the literature and find that the records show that in one case in every one thousand children who receive this particular injection, there is a mild reaction.

What would you tell the mother about the chance of her child suffering a reaction?

Commentary

We are sure that your instinctive response would be to say that the chance of suffering a mild reaction was small. If you used the knowledge you've gained from this unit, you would be able to put a figure on the level of probability one in a thousand, or $\frac{1}{1000}$. The mother could then make up her own mind if she wanted to take this risk.

It would be important to stress to the mother that this low risk does not guarantee that her child would suffer no reaction. Hers could be the one child in a thousand who will – that outcome is *unlikely*, but not impossible.

We also use probability theory in more sophisticated ways as part of everyday life, as the next short activity demonstrates.

ACTIVITY 21

ALLOW 2 MINUTES

Think about your answer to *Activity 20*, where we concluded that the probability of throwing a six at dice was $\frac{1}{6}$. Suppose you shake two dice together – what is the probability of getting a double six? Do you think it is larger or smaller than $\frac{1}{6}$?

Commentary

It is very likely that your natural response to this activity was 'The chance is much less'. You might have a feel for the size of that chance, especially if you play cards or do the pools.

In fact, the answer is one chance in 36 – $\frac{1}{36}$ – which is the result of multiplying together the probabilities of getting a six for each dice.

$\frac{1}{6} \times \frac{1}{6} = \frac{1}{36}$.

Sometimes people wonder why we multiply probabilities when calculating the chance of two random events happening together, rather than adding them. The explanation is as follows.

By the very nature of probability, the probabilities of each of the possible outcomes of a random event add up to 1. So when rolling a dice, there are six possible outcomes, each of which has a probability of ⅙.

Now, when we roll two dice together there are a lot more possible outcomes. We could get a double six, a double five, a one and a three, and so on. If you made a list of all the different ways in which two dice could fall – all of them equally probable – you would find that there are 36. So the probability of any one of these is 1/36. This is the same as multiplying the chances of any two of them happening together.

Armed with this knowledge, it is quite easy to calculate the probability of any number of random events happening together. For example, the chance of throwing a triple six with any one roll of three dice is ⅙ x ⅙ x ⅙. This is a long shot, but it does happen.

We don't need to pursue the maths any further. The understanding you now have about random events is quite sufficient as a basis for studying how genetic predictions can be made.

We'll begin by considering the way that the sex of a baby is determined and the characteristics which are associated with that event. But first, let's summarise the previous few pages.

Summary of Section 1

- Random events happen without any clear pattern; there is no single cause.

- The world is full of random events, and we have an intuitive understanding of what they are.

- The chance of a particular outcome of a random event is expressed as a fraction. One chance in two is the same as ½ or one half.

- The chance of two independent random events occurring together is obtained by multiplying their separate chances together.

2: The determination of sex

Sometimes parents and health professionals are very anxious to know the sex of the baby. There are all kinds of reasons for this, including the fact that some illnesses are sex-linked.

ACTIVITY 22 ALLOW 15 MINUTES

We have already mentioned one disease – haemophilia – which is associated with the sex of the child. Check back over the work you have done so far, and take another look at *Resource 4*. Can you identify any other sex-linked conditions? Make a note of them below.

Commentary

Sex-linked conditions include classical haemophilia, Duchenne muscular dystrophy and a number of other conditions which are relatively rare but serious, such as the Fragile X syndrome mentioned in *Resource 4*.

In families with a history of such a condition it is possible to predict the chance that a male baby will be affected by the illness.

So the sex of a new baby is the outcome of a random event which may be of great importance. Let's look at how it comes about.

The sex chromosomes

Like all of a person's characteristics, sex is determined by the genetic code in the fertilised egg. The information which makes one person male and another female is contained in the genes and located on the chromosomes.

Therefore, we would expect to find differences in the chromosomes in male and female cells. Earlier (in *Figure 8*) you studied a display of human chromosomes and saw that the complete set consisted of 46 chromosomes, constituting 23 pairs. This number is found in all the cells of the body (the **somatic** cells). It is termed the **diploid** number of chromosomes. Each animal and plant species has its own characteristic number.

- In human female cells, all the pairs consist of twin chromosomes,

but

- In human male cells, one of the pairs is made up of two chromosomes which don't match – one is much smaller than the other. This is the pair which carries the genes determining sex, and they are therefore called the sex chromosomes.

The sex chromosomes are identified by the letters X and Y. All male cells have one X and one smaller Y – XY. Female cells have no Y chromosomes; they have two Xs – XX.

As far as we can tell, the differences between males and females arise from the fact that males have this smaller Y chromosome instead of a second X. This can be deduced from the study of people who have somehow inherited the wrong number of sex chromosomes.

People with an extra X chromosome – XXX – or with only one X – XO – are female. People with an extra Y – XYY – are male. There are no cases of living people without an X chromosome at all – YO. So it seems that everyone must have at least one X, but the addition of a Y chromosome always results in maleness.

The Y chromosome is relatively small and very few genes have yet been located on it. However, we know that it bears one called the **testes determining factor (TDF) gene**.

In the early weeks of embryonic life, all embryos show the same development of their early sex organs. At about six weeks in male embryos, the TDF gene is somehow switched on and the primitive sex organs start to turn into testes. The embryo is then committed to male development.

These facts about sex chromosomes raise many questions about the biological nature of maleness and femaleness. They have given rise to heated arguments about the superiority of one sex or the other. I don't intend to enter into these debates in this unit. Instead, in the next section, we will consider how differences in the genetic make-up of male and female cells arise.

Summary of Section 2

- The human nucleus contains 23 pairs of chromosomes (the diploid number of chromosomes).

- One pair, the sex chromosomes, govern the development of sexual characteristics.

- The members of this pair are termed the X and Y chromosomes. Females have two Xs, males have one X and one Y.

- The possession of the Y chromosome determines maleness.

- On the Y chromosome is the TDF gene, which is responsible for the early embryo switching over to development as a male.

3: Formation of eggs and sperm

Reduction division

In Session One, I described the process of mitosis. This results in the production of daughter cells with the same number and type of chromosomes as their parent. If the sex cells were formed by the same process there would be a problem when the egg and sperm united at conception. The fertilised egg would have twice the normal complement of genetic material and twice the normal number of chromosomes.

This situation is avoided because a different method of cell division is used for the production of eggs and sperm. The method results in the number of chromosomes in the sex cells being *half* the normal number. It is called reduction division, or **meiosis**. *Figure 10* shows the nucleus of a cell undergoing this process. Before studying this you might like to look again at Activity 14, where you worked through the process taking place during mitosis. This will help you to see how the two types of cell division compare.

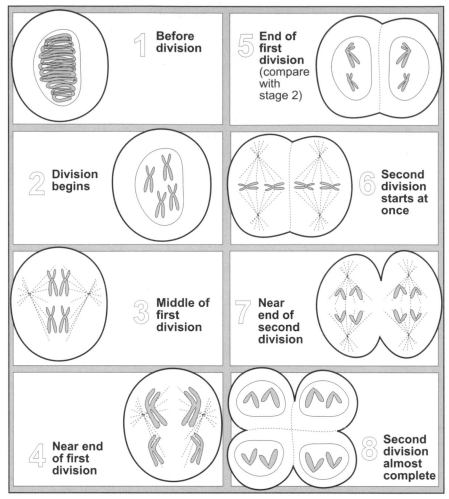

Figure 10 Meiosis: the process of 'reduction division'
(Two pairs of chromosomes only are shown in this diagram)

ACTIVITY 23

Study *Figure 10* and then, in your own words, write a description of what is happening. Make a note of the main differences between this process and mitotic cell division.

Commentary

You may have noticed that, just as in mitosis, the chromosomes appear as double structures and line up across the middle of the cell. However, in meiosis they line up *in pairs* (Frame 3) and, instead of the double chromosomes splitting to begin with, the pairs separate to produce two daughter cells, each with half the usual number of double chromosomes (Frame 6).

Next, these daughter cells themselves divide. The second part of reduction division is just the same as mitosis. The double chromosomes line up across the middle of each daughter cell nucleus and split. The result is four new nuclei, each with half the number of chromosomes found in the rest of the body cells (Frame 8). The number is termed the **haploid** number.

As far as the *nucleus* is concerned, this process occurs in the same way in the formation of both eggs and sperm. There are differences in the way that the rest of the cell's material is divided up. This is because the sperm contains very little beside the nucleus, whereas the egg contains a large food reserve. However, these differences are not relevant here; we are concerned only with what is taking place in the nucleus.

Many of the events in the nucleus have the characteristics of random events. When the pairs of chromosomes line up across the middle of the nucleus it is pure chance which way up any pair may lie. So when they separate the way that the chromosomes are dealt out to the daughter cells is again a matter of chance. These random events really are like shuffling and dealing a hand of cards. The daughter cells each get a different mixture (their 'hand') from the parents' 'pack'.

Male or female sperm

During meiosis, the sex chromosomes behave like all the other pairs. Let's consider what this means for the formation of sex cells. First of all, the production of sperm.

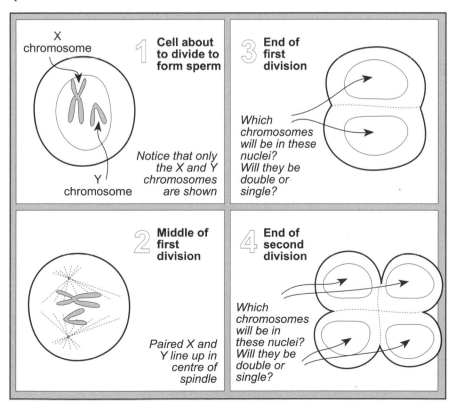

Figure 11 The behaviour of X and Y chromosomes during meiosis in the cells of the testes

ACTIVITY 24   ALLOW 10 MINUTES

Figure 11 represents only the sex chromosomes. Don't forget that there are 22 other pairs also taking part in the process.

See if you can complete the third and fourth frames of the diagram, to show how the X and Y chromosomes will be distributed to the four daughter nuclei. How many of these will contain a Y chromosome?

Commentary

If you followed the pattern of *Figure 10*, your diagram should have shown you that two sperm nuclei will each contain a Y chromosome. The other two will each contain an X. As this will happen in all the sperm-producing cells in the same way, half the total sperm cells produced will contain a Y chromosome and the other half an X chromosome.

Knowing that it is the possession of a Y chromosome which determines maleness, we can call the Y-containing sperm 'male sperm'. There is a ½ chance of any particular sperm being male.

As far as we know, neither male nor female sperm have any advantage when fertilisation occurs. In each ejaculate, there are at least 250 million sperm cells. A high proportion of them are defective in some way, possibly because the wearing of clothes by human beings raises the temperature in the testes where they are formed. There does not seem to be any difference, however, between abnormalities in male and female sperm, although there is a great deal still to be learnt about this topic.

In the present state of knowledge it is safe to say that the chance of an egg being fertilised by either an X- or a Y-containing sperm is the same. So, at every conception, the sex of the baby is essentially a matter of chance.

Summary of Section 3

- Sex cells (eggs and sperm) are formed by meiosis, a process of reduction-division which occurs only in the formation of sex cells.
- During the first part of this process, the double chromosomes line up along the middle of the spindle in pairs.
- Each pair then separates producing two daughter nuclei, each with the haploid number of double chromosomes.
- This is the first division of meiosis. It does not occur in mitosis.
- A second division then starts at once.
- This is just the same as mitosis. The double chromosomes line up (unpaired) across the middle of the spindle.
- They then split and the two halves separate.
- The end result is four new nuclei, each with the haploid number of single chromosomes.
- So meiosis is a process in which the DNA replicates once, but the nucleus divides twice.
- During meiotic division, random events lead to a shuffling of the chromosomes so that sex cells get different combinations from the parent cells.
- The sex chromosomes behave in exactly the same way as other chromosomes during meiosis and mitosis.

- There is a ½ chance that any particular egg will be fertilised by a Y-containing sperm. Therefore, at each conception, there is a ½ chance that the baby will be a boy.

4: Random mistakes

In describing meiosis and the contribution which it makes to variation, I have talked about the situation where everything happens as it should. However, in the series of random events which occur when the chromosomes are shuffled around before they divide, there are many opportunities for things to go wrong. When this happens, the chromosomes are not distributed correctly and the result is a chromosomal abnormality. A cell may end up with an extra chromosome, or part of a chromosome may remain attached to its partner after they separate.

You have probably come across people with learning difficulties who are affected by Down syndrome. These people have an extra copy of chromosome 21 – one of the smallest of the chromosomes. They therefore have 47 chromosomes in all.

ACTIVITY 25   ALLOW **15** MINUTES

Now I would like you to read *Resource 5*, which describes the features of Down syndrome.

As you read, note down the systems affected by the presence of this small extra chromosome.

Commentary

Perhaps you have observed that Down syndrome is related to particular changes in:

- the musculoskeletal system
- the teeth
- the skin.

These changes give rise to some of the external features which can be observed.

There are also effects in:

- the heart
- the digestive system
- the renal system

- the hormonal system
- the reproductive system.

People with Down syndrome show certain disabilities and personality traits too, so the effects of this extra chromosome are very wide ranging.

The metaphor of a book that I have been using up to now would not help to explain why the presence of one small 'chapter' should alter the contents of the entire volume. We need to look at this in more detail.

5: A question of balance

The relationship between the different sections of the genetic material is not very well understood at present. However, it appears that 'normal' development depends on a state of balance between all of the genetic material in a person's cells. In some way that we don't yet understand, the parts of the code interact to produce normal growth and development. So the tiny extra chromosome in a person with Down syndrome alters the balance and changes most of the genetic instructions which govern the body systems.

The question of balance between all the parts of the genetic material is of fundamental importance. Here is the point where our metaphor of a 'book' breaks down, since we do not know of any book in which the chapters interact.

However, the idea of the book has been useful up to this point as a way of demonstrating the various levels of organisation of the genetic material. We can use this to look at the way in which the totality of a person's genetic code balances out to produce observable characters. In other words, we shall look at patterns of inheritance.

Summary of Sections 4 and 5

- Random events during meiosis can result in a faulty distribution of the chromosomes to produce a chromosomal abnormality in the egg or sperm which will be passed on to the fertilised egg and therefore to the next generation.

- Down syndrome is a condition in which a small extra chromosome is passed on in this way.

- Down syndrome produces wide-ranging and characteristic effects, some advantageous and some disadvantageous.

- 'Normal' development from a fertilised egg appears to depend on a state of balance between all parts of the genome.

6: Sex-linked characteristics

I would like to start this section by thinking about the balance between the two sex chromosomes.

You have seen that the Y chromosome is small and appears to bear few genes in comparison with the X. It is known to bear the TDF gene which initiates male development in the embryo, and is responsible for the primary and secondary sexual characteristics which relate to the male reproductive system.

Some conditions that we have already studied are clearly linked to sex; for example, haemophilia and Duchenne muscular dystrophy are confined to men. It would be logical to suppose that these conditions are determined by genes on the sex chromosomes, and this is indeed the case.

Haemophilia is a good example of the pattern of inheritance. There are several kinds of haemophilia. Each is caused by a deficiency in one of the factors responsible for normal blood clotting. The type I will consider here is classical haemophilia – or haemophilia A – which results from the deficiency of Factor VIII, a protein which plays an essential part in the clotting of blood.

ACTIVITY 26   ALLOW 5 MINUTES

Take a few moments to review what you have already learnt concerning this illness and its pattern of inheritance.

Commentary

In Session One you saw how the condition affected Queen Victoria's family. All affected individuals were male and the condition appeared to be passed from one generation to another via 'carrier' females. (I will explain the technical meaning of 'carrier' shortly.)

The gene which controls the production of Factor VIII is found on the X chromosome. If it is faulty, this protein will not be manufactured, so normal blood clotting won't take place. Even a minor trauma will damage blood vessels and lead to prolonged blood loss.

Every cell (except the sex cells) has two sets of genes on the two sets of chromosomes, one of which comes from the mother and one from the father. All women have two X chromosomes, and therefore two Factor VIII genes. If one of these genes is faulty, the other one will be able to bring about normal Factor VIII production. So the two genes will balance – one will 'hide' the effect of the other. A woman with a faulty gene will not be affected by haemophilia, but she will be a **carrier** of the faulty gene. A carrier is someone who is able to transmit a disease to others without being affected by it themselves.

In this woman's ovaries, the X chromosome with the faulty gene will be present in half of all the egg cells she produces. The other half will have the normal X chromosome. Since the distribution of the X chromosome to her eggs is a random process, we can make some predictions about the way the faulty gene is passed to her children.

ALLOW **10** MINUTES

Let's consider the next egg that this carrier woman is going to liberate from her ovaries. Suppose that it is one with a faulty Factor VIII gene and it is fertilised by sperm from a partner who has a normal Factor VIII gene. *Figure 12* shows the possible outcomes of this event.

Study *Figure 12* carefully. Notice that instead of using pictures, I have shown the chromosomes as letters.

X_H= an X chromosome with the faulty gene (causing haemophilia)
X_N= an X chromosome with a normal copy of the gene
Y= the Y chromosome

Now study the diagram and fill in the blank spaces in the box below it.

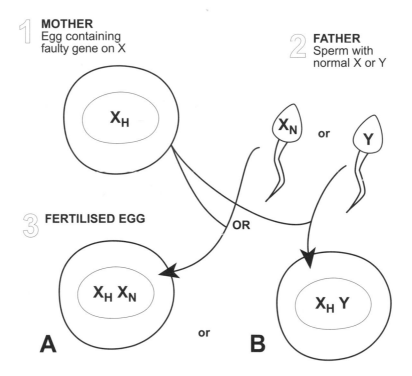

Figure 12 The impact of the faulty gene

The resulting baby will be either:

	Sex?		Carrier or sufferer?
1	A	who is a	of haemophilia
or			
2	A	who is a	of haemophilia

1   Because the process of fertilisation is, as far as we can tell, a random one, all the sperm have an equal chance of getting to fertilise the egg. So there is a ½ chance that the one that does succeed contains an X chromosome.

If this happens, the resulting baby will be female. She will have one normal X chromosome, so the effect of the faulty Factor VIII gene will be masked. She will *not* be affected by the illness. She will, however, have one copy of the faulty gene, which will make her a carrier of the illness.

2   There is also a ½ chance that the sperm that reaches the target contains a Y chromosome. In this case, the baby will be male. He will have only one X chromosome, bearing a faulty Factor VIII gene. He will not be able to produce Factor VIII; therefore, he *will* suffer from haemophilia.

The carrier state for this and many other genetically determined diseases can now be identified by blood tests. Let's see what predictions could be made about a carrier woman's children, and consider what advice she might be given.

ACTIVITY 28   ALLOW **10** MINUTES

1   Draw a diagram to show what will happen to the X chromosomes in this person's ovarian cells during the formation of egg cells. Use the pattern shown in *Figure 11* to help here.

2   What is the chance that the next egg cell she produces will contain a faulty Factor VIII gene?

3   If the egg is fertilised by a sperm from an unaffected partner, what is the chance that it will meet a Y-containing sperm?

4   As a result of your answers to questions 2 and 3, what do you think is the chance of the conception we are considering producing an affected male child? Look back to *Activity 21* to help with the answer.

Commentary

1   Here is a diagram to show what will happen to the X chromosomes.

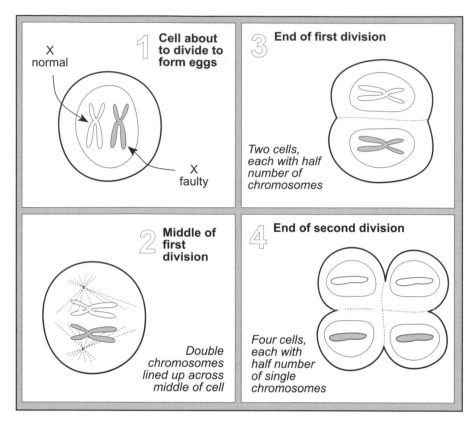

Figure 13 The distribution of X chromosomes in the eggs of a woman who carries the faulty gene causing haemophilia

So the end result of each division is four potential egg cells. Two will have the normal X chromosome and two will have the faulty one. In fact, only one of the four grows to become an egg, but which one grows is purely a matter of chance.

2 The chance of her next egg cell containing a faulty Factor VIII gene is ½. This is apparent from the diagram.

3 The chance of the egg being fertilised by a Y-containing sperm is also ½.

4 Building on these answers, and from the principles set out in *Activity 21*, you will probably have decided that the chance of these two random events happening together is ½ x ½ = ¼. So there is a one in four chance that the next child this woman conceives will be an affected male.

Predictions of this kind can be made for any characteristic which is affected by a single gene on any of the chromosomes, not just the sex chromosomes. They can be made *because* the processes of cell division and fertilisation are random events.

This applies to characteristics, like illness, where the gene is either faulty or normal, and also to characteristics where there are alternative forms of 'normal', as you will see in the next section.

Summary of Section 6

- The different parts of the genetic material do not work in isolation. They interact in ways that are not fully understood at present.

- Normal development depends on the balance between all the parts of the genetic material.

- The sex chromosomes bear some genes which are not concerned with sexual development. They are responsible for sex-linked characteristics.

- Some of the genes on the X chromosome are responsible for serious illnesses, such as haemophilia and Duchenne muscular dystrophy.

- Because women have two X chromosomes, a faulty gene on one X will be balanced by a normal gene on the other.

- Because men have only one X chromosome, the effects of a faulty gene on the X chromosome will be evident.

7: Clear-cut inheritance patterns

As we have just seen, a female carrier of haemophilia has two different copies of the Factor VIII gene – one normal and one faulty. The faulty one is 'hidden' by the effects of the corresponding normal gene. Such genes are termed **recessive**. They will only show up in the absence of a normal gene, so we have a situation where some people with the gene are affected and others are carriers.

Other faulty genes always show up, even if the partner chromosome has a normal gene. These are called **dominant** genes. All individuals with the gene are affected.

The serious disabling condition **Huntington's chorea** is an example of the results of a dominant faulty gene. In this condition, people with the faulty gene are perfectly well until late middle age. They then become affected by paralysis and uncontrollable muscular spasms which eventually lead to the loss of movement, speech and the ability to care for themselves.

The set of genes that a person possesses is termed the **genotype**. If both the copies of a given gene in a person's cells are the same, the person is said to have a **homozygous** genotype for that particular characteristic. On the other hand, if the two copies are different, the genotype is **heterozygous**.

So a female carrier of haemophilia has a heterozygous genotype for the Factor VIII gene; a person affected by Huntington's chorea has a heterozygous genotype for the HC gene and a person unaffected by this condition has a homozygous genotype for the HC gene.

The way that the genes are expressed is shown by the way that a particular genotype affects a person's characteristics. The observed effect is termed the **phenotype**. A person who is a carrier for haemophilia has a **normal** phenotype, whereas a person who has the illness shows the **affected** phenotype.

For many genes there are not just two alternative forms. There may be more than two although a person's cells will contain only two. This gives rise to a wider range of different genotypes and therefore more than two possible phenotypes. This is clearly shown in a case of considerable interest to nurses: a person's blood group.

Blood groups

The set of genes that determines a person's blood group has been intensively studied. Blood collected from healthy donors must be acceptable in the body of the recipient. Doctors who tried to transfuse blood in the early days soon found that there were differences in the blood of healthy people. This led to an active search for the sources of this variation and to the discovery of the various blood grouping systems in use today.

These systems are just ways of describing the differences in the surface proteins of normal blood cells.

Blood consists of a fluid part, the **plasma**, in which several kinds of blood cells are suspended. There are the **white cells**, which are part of the body's defence mechanism – the immune system – and the **red cells**, which carry oxygen combined with haemoglobin. The red cells are surrounded by an outer membrane which is partly composed of proteins. The ones on the outside of the membrane are the **surface proteins**. They function as part of the structure of the cell and they are rather like its 'face', since they can be recognised by the immune system.

This system is geared up to attack any foreign protein from outside the body as this could be on the surface of a disease-causing bacterium. So there are no questions asked when a foreign protein enters the body, even if it is on an otherwise harmless blood cell from another person.

Each type of surface protein is controlled by its particular gene. These genes exist in alternative forms. The consequences of these variations are not detrimental. They produce normal, but slightly different, alternative forms of the surface proteins.

The first set of these proteins to be discovered were those of the ABO blood group. These are governed by three alternative forms of one particular gene on chromosome 9.

Now we know that each person has two copies of chromosome 9, and therefore two copies of this gene. But the gene can exist in three alternative forms. In the next activity, you can work out for yourself how the ABO blood groups arise.

ACTIVITY 29 — ALLOW 3 MINUTES

Using the information which you have just considered, work out all the possible combinations of two genes from the set of three – A, B and O.

List these in the first column of the following table, headed Genetic make-up. For example, you may choose two As for the first combination, and write 'AA' in the table (as in the example entry) and A plus O for the second, which you would note down as AO.

For the moment, you need only complete the first column.

You will be able to review your answer when you have completed the table during the next activity.

1 Genetic make-up	2 Blood group	3 Antibodies in the blood	4 Transfusion of cells from—
AA	A	B	A & O

Table 2 ABO blood groups

When blood transfusions were first tried, the recipients often suffered a severe reaction. In the laboratory it was seen that the red cells in the donor's blood were often affected when mixed with the recipient's blood. They were first clumped together and then destroyed.

The donor red cells were being treated as foreign bodies by the fluid part of the recipient's blood. Later it was discovered that the recipient's plasma was producing antibodies against the surface proteins of donor red cells. Two proteins, A and B, caused the recipient to produce anti A and anti B antibodies.

Clearly, if someone has the A protein on their blood cells, their immune system will not attack it, as it won't be foreign to their body. They will not make the anti A antibody.

Conversely, if they *do not* have A on their own cells, they *will* make anti A, as A is a foreign protein. Using this information, you will be able to work out the antibody responses which people of different genetic make-up can produce.

ACTIVITY 30   ALLOW 10 MINUTES

1   A person's blood group is described as A, B, AB or O. Group A people have only A surface protein; group B have only B; group AB have both and group O have neither.

Look back to *Table 2*, and fill in the second column showing the blood groups for the genetic types in the first column. We have completed the first line of the table as an example, showing that a person with genetic make-up AA, having only A surface proteins, must be blood group A. (Note that some of the genetic types you have included will produce the same blood group.)

2   Next, for each of the blood groups, work out which antibodies they can produce in their own plasma, and complete the third column. Our example shows that people with blood group A will have B antibodies in their blood.

3   Finally, think about the kind of red blood cells which could be given by transfusion to people with each of these blood groups. Remember that it is only safe to transfuse red cells if the recipient does not have antibodies to attack their surface proteins.

Record your answers in the fourth column. The example entry shows that people with B antibodies can receive blood only from people without B surface proteins.

Now compare your answers with those I have provided below in *Table 3*.

1 Genetic make-up	2 Blood group	3 Antibodies in the blood	4 Transfusion of cells from—
AA	A	B	A & O
AB	AB	None	A, B, AB & O
AO	A	B	A & O
BB	B	A	B & O
BO	B	A	B & O
OO	O	AB	O

Table 3 ABO blood groups: the completed table

Commentary

From this table you will see that, in theory, blood group O can be given to people with any blood group. However, the picture is not quite so simple, because there are several other sets of surface proteins which give rise to other blood grouping systems. For safe transfusion, patient and donor blood must be matched to the fullest possible extent.

This is why, prior to transfusion, various tests are done on donor and recipient blood, including cross-matching in which a sample of the recipient's plasma is tested directly with the donor cells. If the recipient's plasma contains antibodies against any of the surface proteins on the donor's cells, it will cause them to clump together. This effect is quickly and easily seen in the laboratory.

When caring for a patient having a blood transfusion, nurses and midwives look out for certain physical signs. These are the result of reactions between the recipient's antibodies and the donor red cells, which are clumped together and then destroyed.

The pattern in which the genes governing the ABO proteins are passed from parent to child is very clear. If a person has the genetic make-up AA – and is therefore blood group A – they have received one A gene from the father and one A gene from the mother. Therefore, both that person's parents must have had at least one A gene. Their father couldn't be blood group B or O. This pattern is the basis on which it is possible to make some statements about the relationships between parents and children – which can be significant in cases where this relationship is in dispute.

The inheritance pattern is also very important in relation to the blood groups of a mother and her unborn baby. The baby's red cells come into contact with the mother's blood in the placenta at the time of birth, but not before. If the two kinds of blood are incompatible, the mother's immune system will make antibodies against the baby's surface proteins as soon as their bloods come into contact – that is, when the baby is born. This doesn't upset the new baby, because the antibodies develop slowly over the course of a few days after the birth. However, these antibodies can persist until the mother is pregnant again.

If the antibodies persist and the next baby is like the first one, the mother's antibodies will attack the blood of the unborn baby, leading to symptoms which vary from mild to very severe. In the most severe cases, the baby will be stillborn or suffer from haemolytic disease of the newborn (HDN).

The antibodies to the ABO system proteins do not cause very many problems of this kind – which is just as well, because many mothers carry babies of non-compatible ABO blood groups.

However, one of the other blood groups – **the Rhesus (Rh) group** – does cause problems. A severe reaction occurs when a mother without the Rh factor has antibodies to the Rh protein and is pregnant with a child who has inherited the Rh factor from its father – in other words, when an Rh negative woman is pregnant with an Rh positive baby.

A first Rh pregnancy is usually trouble-free, but after the birth the mother's blood is ready to attack any future Rh positive baby, and subsequent pregnancies may be severely affected. Fortunately, this can now be prevented by giving any Rh negative mother bearing an Rh positive first baby artificial protection from the baby's blood cells at the time of its birth. This is given by an injection which wipes out any of the baby's cells which have leaked into the mother's blood before they can stimulate her immune system to produce antibodies. This relatively simple procedure has reduced the incidence of HDN dramatically.

You may have noticed that, in the case of blood groups, the differences between people are very clear-cut. A person is either Rh positive or Rh negative, they suffer from haemophilia or they do not. Situations like this arise where a characteristic is controlled by a single gene and its various alternative forms.

In practice, however, most of the characteristics we observe are not like this. If you look back at your observations in *Activity 4*, you will see that it is difficult to put people into clearly defined categories. We can say that people are fat or thin, tall or short ... but where exactly do we draw the line between these categories?

Characteristics like this are said to be **continuously varying**. They are the product of genes acting together, and their patterns of inheritance are therefore much more complex than those for single genes.

We will consider characteristics of this type in the next section.

Summary of Section 7

- Some alternative forms of any gene are recessive. They show up only if they are not balanced out by another form of the gene.

- Some alternative forms are dominant. They always show up.

- The ABO blood grouping system is based on three alternative forms of a single gene.

- The alternative forms of the protein produced by the gene are responsible for antibody production and can thus give rise to a transfusion reaction if donor and recipient blood are not compatible.

- The Rhesus blood group antibodies can produce a severe reaction in an Rh negative mother who becomes pregnant with a second Rh positive baby.

- Blood group proteins show clear-cut inheritance patterns because they are controlled by single-gene systems.

8: Continuous variation

A person's body height is a characteristic which can vary from very short to very tall, with all the possible values in between. We could use height as an example to explore the inheritance of continuously varying characteristics. However, for practical purposes, it is easier to use another measure of body configuration – shoe size.

ACTIVITY 31   ALLOW 30 MINUTES

Collect shoe sizes from as many adult people, either men or women, as you possibly can. Aim for fifty or more – this is why I said it would be helpful to work with a colleague. Don't use a mixture of men and women; stick to one or the other.

Make a list of the sizes. This is your raw data. Looking at the list, you will probably find it difficult to see any pattern. So I would like you to arrange the data in such a way that, if there is a pattern, it will be clear.

The best way to do this is to arrange the data in categories of ascending size. You could group sizes and half-sizes together to give the categories shown in the first column of *Table 4*.

For this activity, collect your data over a few days, and then allow about 30 minutes to prepare the chart. You can work either alone or with a colleague or a group of colleagues.

1 Shoe size	2 Number of people
$2 - 2^1/_2$	
$3 - 3^1/_2$	
$4 - 4^1/_2$	
$5 - 5^1/_2$	
$6 - 6^1/_2$	
$7 - 7^1/_2$	
$8 - 8^1/_2$	
$9 - 9^1/_2$	
$10 - 10^1/_2$	
$11 - 11^1/_2$	
$12 - 12^1/_2$	

Table 4 Shoe sizes

Go through your list of raw data and, for each shoe size that you have collected, put a cross in the second column against the appropriate category.

When you have completed *Table 4*, turn the page round until the first column is horizontal at its lower edge. You will find that you now have a bar-chart of the distribution of shoe sizes for your group of people.

Note down anything that interests you about the shape that has been created.

Commentary

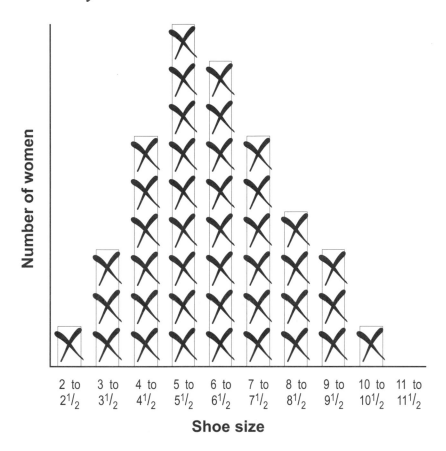

Figure 14 A bar-chart for women's shoe sizes

Figure 14 shows a typical example of the kind of chart you might have compiled. The things you might have noted include:

1   The chart shows that there are some people with shoe sizes in most of the categories.

2   There is a normal range of values. Few adults have shoe size less than 3 or greater than 12.

3   Most women have a shoe size somewhere in the middle of the normal range.

4   The chart you have drawn shows a single peak. If you had collected your data from a mixed group of men and women, you would have found two distinct peaks because most men have larger shoe sizes than most women.

The chart you have drawn may not look exactly like *Figure 14* because by chance you may have picked a sample of people with rather large or rather small feet. This is perfectly possible. However, if you collected a lot more shoe sizes to add to the chart, you would find in the end that the shape in *Figure 14* would begin to emerge.

The shape shown by the bar-chart is called a **Gaussian distribution**. It is a bell-like shape and describes the distribution of many other continuously varying characteristics, for example, height and weight. This kind of curve is a sign that the characteristic is the product of several genes acting together, and the effects of the environment, too. So in the case of humans, we wouldn't expect to find a single 'tallness' gene, but several acting together to determine an individual person's genetic potential in terms of height. The attainment of that potential would then depend upon environmental factors, such as adequate nutrition.

It follows from this that we cannot make precise predictions about the characteristics of the offspring based on those of the parents. All the genes involved are subject to the same random events, but the mathematics is no longer simple. We can be certain that the children of tall parents are more likely to inherit some of the 'tallness' genes than are children of short parents, but we can't say how likely it is.

Selective breeding

People who breed plants and animals make use of these tendencies to carry out selective breeding programmes to encourage desired characteristics. So we get roses with bigger and better flowers and fewer thorns by breeding from the largest and least thorny parents, for example.

Selective human breeding has been advocated in the past, with terrible consequences during the second World War when Hitler tried to wipe out the non-Aryan races and encourage the breeding of a 'pure' Aryan people.

Policies such as this are repugnant to us today, but questions arise as more advances are made in reproductive technology. For example, Artificial Insemination by Donor (AID) is now a realistic option and there have been suggestions that women should be able to choose an AID donor for his desirable mental or physical characteristics. Questions like this are outside the scope of this unit, but if you are interested you can read more about them in the sources given in the Further Reading section.

In the last two sections we have seen that in a relatively few cases, a characteristic can be directly related to the alternative forms of a single gene and show clear-cut patterns of inheritance. Most characteristics are governed by the interaction of several genes and the effect of the environment on the way that they are expressed. This gives rise to the continuous variation which we can observe.

However, this is still not the end of the story. There are two more sources of variation, two more sets of random events, which we need to consider before we have the complete picture. But first, here is a summary of the main points of this section.

Summary of Section 8

- Many characteristics that we observe do not show clear-cut inheritance patterns.

- These characteristics result from the interaction of several genes and the environment.

- In the population, these characteristics tend to show a Gaussian distribution.

9: Still more variation

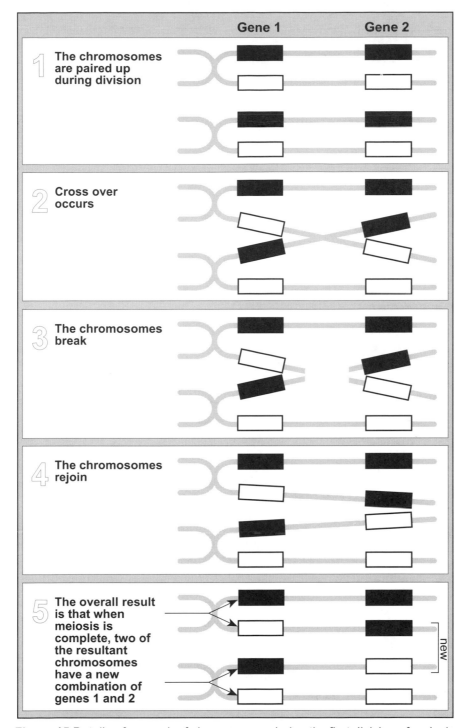

| Gene 1 | Gene 2 |

1 The chromosomes are paired up during division

2 Cross over occurs

3 The chromosomes break

4 The chromosomes rejoin

5 The overall result is that when meiosis is complete, two of the resultant chromosomes have a new combination of genes 1 and 2

new

Figure 15 Details of one pair of chromosomes during the first division of meiosis

The first of the two remaining sources of variation is a process that occurs during the formation of eggs and sperms. It takes place during meiosis, during the first division, when the double chromosomes line up in pairs along the spindle. You might like to review Section 3 to remind yourself how this takes place. Then go back to look at *Figure 15*, which provides more details of what happens to the chromosomes.

In this diagram the chromosomes are shown as lines, for the sake of clarity. The location of two genes (genes 1 and 2) is shown by boxes and the alternative forms of each of these genes are shown as either black or white boxes.

Figure 15 shows what happens. You should note that one pair of double chromosomes is shown here in diagrammatic form.

ACTIVITY 32

Study *Figure 15* and write a short account, in your own words, of what appears to be taking place in this dividing nucleus.

Commentary

Figure 15 shows what happens to one pair of chromosomes during meiosis – remember that there are 22 other pairs. An account of what is happening goes something like this:

The first frame of the diagram shows a pair of double chromosomes next to each other. For some reason, two bits of the chromosomes next to each other seem to cross over. They are then exchanged so that each chromosome has a bit of its partner. On these chromosomes, genes 1 and 2 are shown. The result of this exchange process is that each chromosome now has a different combination of the forms of the first and second genes.

Let's expand on this explanation.

When meiosis begins, the chromosomes double and pair up, as we have already seen. This happens during the process of coiling and thickening which is necessary in order to organise the long DNA threads so that they can be shared out equally to the daughter nuclei. In fact, the coiled chromosomes are about 700 times thicker than the unwound DNA, so you can imagine how much coiling and folding occurs.

During the coiling and thickening, it sometimes happens by chance – a random event – that the ends of the paired chromosomes get wrapped around each other. If this occurs, the chromosomes may be put under such strain that they break momentarily.

After a break, the ends rejoin, but not always at the right place – they may become joined to their partner. Thus the partner chromosomes exchange sections. The process of exchange is known as **crossing over**.

The process of crossing over results in the alternative forms of the genes occurring in new combinations in the sex cells formed. It is an extremely important way of producing variety within families. Without it, children would be much more like their parents than they are.

Although crossing over is a random event, we can be certain about some aspects of its occurrence, and this is helpful to scientists who are studying the human genetic map. It is clear that the chance of a break occurring between two genes which are very close together is much less than the chance of it happening between those which are far apart. So characteristics which always show up together are likely to be governed by genes close together on the same chromosomes.

This fact helps in the process of mapping the human genome. This is not just a theoretical exercise but has many practical applications. For example, there are some faulty genes which cannot be detected directly in the cell. The gene responsible for Huntington's chorea is one of these. However, it is known that another gene which is detectable always occurs with the Huntington's chorea gene. It is therefore called a **marker gene** and it can be used to detect the presence of the faulty gene before its effects are felt.

The second remaining cause of variation is mutation, an actual change in a gene which may produce recognisable phenotype effects. This, too, is a random event. Since we will be looking at mutation in some detail in Session Four, I will say little about it here except that it provides the source of new, alternative forms of the genes.

The overall effect of all the random genetic events described in this section is that many of our observable characteristics are distributed in the same way as shoe size. If you were to repeat *Activity 31* measuring weight, blood pressure or serum glucose you would get a chart with a similar shape. The measurements in the centre are those that we tend to think of as 'normal' values.

What is 'normal'?

It is common practice in health care to refer to a 'normal range of values' for various things that can be measured. If a measurement falls outside that range, a health problem is suspected.

For example, the height and weight of children in their early years are provided in the form of **centile charts** which show the 'normal' range of values at various ages. These charts show the way in which children normally grow and it is possible to plot the growth rate of a baby on the chart and compare it with the normal rate of progress.

If the measurements of a baby fall below this range on several occasions, then there is concern that the baby may not be thriving. It is quite possible that this particular baby is normally small, but care must be taken to ensure that there is no other reason for the observations.

This example shows how difficult it is to decide what is 'normal' and what constitutes a health problem. In Session Three, we'll look at the way what we call normal has been developed as the human race has evolved.

Summary of Section 9

- Most of our physical and mental characteristics are governed by several genes acting together.

- They do not all show clear cut patterns of inheritance.

- Characters like this often show a Gaussian distribution when we study them in large numbers of people.

- Two sources of variation are the exchange of sections of chromosomes – crossing over – which takes place during meiosis, and changes in the genes themselves – mutations.

- The result of all these random sources of variation is the establishment of 'normal' values for the characteristics of human beings.

Let's end this second section by applying the principles we have considered to people needing care. Let's take another look at the subject of one of our case studies and revise the random genetic events that have happened in her life.

10: Looking at patients and clients

Take a moment or two to go back and read over the case study I presented earlier, in Session One, pages 36 and 37. This sets out the details leading up to Mary's diagnosis and treatment for carcinoma of the breast. I would like you to use it to revise the work you have done in this session.

ACTIVITY 33   ALLOW 5 MINUTES

Like everyone else, Mary's genetic history will have contained many random events. Think about her life from the time that the egg from which she grew was formed in her mother's ovary. Make a list of the random genetic events which must have happened from that time up to the present.

Commentary

1   This egg must have been formed by meiosis (reduction/division). This involved the following random events:

- the way that the double chromosomes lined up at the start of cell division
- crossing over at this stage
- the way that the chromosomes were distributed to daughter cells.

2   We know that, in this process, the chromosome bearing the early-onset cancer gene ended up in the nucleus of the egg that was to become Mary. When this egg was fertilised, chance alone determined which one of her father's sperm was successful.

3   Then the egg started to grow into Mary and, as she grew and developed, random 'mistakes' could occur each time a cell divided.

4   As Mary's ovaries started to produce eggs, reduction division – with all its random events – happened each time an egg was formed.

Listing all these events for a single person may help to emphasise just how widespread these random processes are. One might imagine that a system which depended on random processes would tend to become disorganised. The amazing thing is that, in the living cell and in living things, we get order rather than chaos. This is one of the great mysteries of modern biology and its solution will be one of the great achievements of science.

What do these ideas offer us in our work as health carers? They provide us with two useful ways of looking at health and illness.

Firstly, they emphasise the random nature of a great deal of ill health that has a genetic basis. There is an inevitability and a lack of any cause about much of what we see and try to help our patients and clients come to terms with.

Secondly, they show how important it is that people are protected from things which increase the number of random genetic mistakes occurring in their bodies. Health carers have an important educative role here, as you will see in Session Four.

In the meantime, I will move on to the next key concept included in this introductory unit: **adaptation**.

You have now reached the end of Session Two. Before you move on to Session Three, check that you have achieved the objectives given at the beginning of this session, and, if not, review the appropriate sections.

SESSION THREE

Adaptation

Overview

The key concepts of variation and randomness which we have discussed so far have supported the view that the variation we see in the human species has arisen from random events which have established our 'normal' characteristics.

In this section, we will be considering why these particular characteristics have been selected as normal. This will introduce the idea of **adaptation** to a particular environment. This is another of the basic ideas which underlies genetics and has also been the inspiration for some of the modern theories of nursing.

I will consider ways in which we are adapted for our environment and what happens when we find ourselves in conditions for which we are not adapted. Then we will think about how modern science helps us to avoid the effects of maladaptation and consider the difficult question of why some maladaptive features persist.

We will end Session Three by applying the theoretical principles which we have developed to the lives of some real people.

Session objectives

When you have completed this session you should be able to:

- explain the advantages for survival of 'normal' characteristics
- give examples of survival behaviour and explain its genetic basis
- outline the effects on health of moving between environments
- make links between the concepts of adaptation and health
- suggest why characteristics may persist despite being unfavourable
- apply these ideas to health-care practice.

Please note this text is written so that it can be understood by people who have not studied genetics at all in the past. It may be you have already achieved these outcomes and wish to use the material for revision purposes.

1: Introducing adaptation

The characteristics which we call 'normal' are so familiar to us that most people never ask the question, 'Why are we like this?'. We take it for granted that most people are of a similar height, somewhere between 1.5 and 2 metres, and that most babies are born at around 40 weeks after conception. What is so special about these particular values?

To begin to explore this question, the next activity asks you to do some more observation on real people – this time on yourself.

ACTIVITY 34   ALLOW 15 MINUTES

To do this activity, you'll need to find a quiet place where you will be undisturbed, and can switch off from the world around you.

Think about your physical self. Starting at your feet and working up, consider each part of your body and see if you can give one good reason for it being just the way it is. For example, if you begin with your toe-nails you might ask, 'What are they for?', 'Do they serve any useful purpose?', 'Why do they keep on growing?', 'What would happen if they weren't there?'.

These questions might lead you to decide that the nails serve a protective function which would be particularly useful if you went barefoot.

Commentary

I wouldn't be surprised if you didn't get very far in ten minutes, because as you thought about your legs and feet you would realise that there is so much to say about them. Our legs are beautifully structured for standing and walking. This is what is meant by adaptation: the human body is adapted for walking upright.

In general, adaptation means being well fitted for a particular way of living and a particular place.

If you got as far as your pelvis, you would observe adaptation for a different purpose. The pelvis serves a number of useful protective and supporting functions. In women, for example, it is broad to allow the passage of a baby's head during childbirth.

Clearly the size of the pelvis influences the structure of the rest of the skeleton. It seems that the human female skeleton is adapted for bearing babies with heads of a particular size.

But you might wonder, why do babies heads have to be that size, and why do they have to have such big heads anyway? Let's explore some answers to these questions.

ACTIVITY 35

When you have some time, discuss with your colleagues and – if possible – an experienced midwife, the reason for babies being the size they are. You will be extending your learning outside the scope of this unit, but this is a good illustration of the way in which the concepts arising in genetics merge with and arc relevant to other aspects of health care.

Commentary

Your discussions may have provided you with some answers that deal with the long pre-natal development of the human baby and the size of the brain at birth. The long period needed for the human brain to mature requires a long period of dependent infancy.

Looking at adaptation in this way tells us that many adaptive features are associated with the birth and survival of the highly dependent infant.

Let's consider this last point in more detail.

2: Adaptation for survival

If the survival of babies is so important to our species, we might expect to find that babies show inborn features that adapt them well for survival. If you have the opportunity to observe a newly-born baby, the next activity will help you to test this idea.

ACTIVITY 36   ALLOW 30 MINUTES

Try to arrange to observe a new baby and its mother for at least half an hour. Note any characteristics which you can observe in both mother and child which would help the child to survive.

Perhaps you could imagine mother and baby cast away on a desert island, with food and water but little in the way of shelter. What characteristics would help the baby survive under these 'natural' conditions?

If you don't have the opportunity to make these observations, talk to someone who has, such as a mother or an experienced midwife.

Commentary

You probably observed or talked about many things which the baby could not possibly have learnt but which contribute to its survival. For instance, nearly all babies are able to suckle right from birth. The way they look is very attractive to adults and arouses protective feelings. They have physiological mechanisms which enable them to survive exposure to cold. Baby and mother interact to form an instinctive bond. The mother establishes lactation in response to the baby's demands. Her physiology becomes adapted to the baby, so that the 'let down' reflex operates when the baby cries with hunger. During pregnancy, the mother stores fat, enabling her to survive difficult conditions and thus support the baby.

In these and lots of other ways, the mother/baby duo shows adaptive features which assist the survival of the child. These have a genetic basis.

As the child grows to adulthood, other adaptive features can be seen. These are the 'echoes' of the characteristics which have contributed to the survival of our ancestors. These days, they are most noticeable at times when personal survival is threatened. The next activity provides an opportunity to see if you can identify some of these characteristics in adults under stress.

ACTIVITY 37 — ALLOW 5 MINUTES

You could carry out this activity in either of two ways, depending on your own experience.

You could think about yourself in difficult circumstances, such as being very cold or short of food or water.

Alternatively, you could think about a patient in severe pain, or someone who has been injured.

Can you identify three things that people do automatically under these circumstances – things which they have not learnt?

1

2

3

Commentary

There are many possible choices, but here are three.

1 When you are very cold, you curl up into a ball. This reduces heat loss, but you don't need to be told to do it – you may not even realise why you are doing it. This would certainly help you survive if you were stranded in the snow.

2 An injured person's body adjusts to cope with blood loss by cutting down the circulation to the skin and concentrating all available blood on the heart and brain. The person looks white and cold, but the chances of survival are increased as long as the brain can be kept going.

3 A person in pain may automatically cry or moan. The survival advantage of this today is not readily apparent, although these noises have a powerful effect on other people who try to help. In earlier times, these cries could have acted as a warning to others or as a means of attracting attention.

None of these things is learnt. They must be present in our genes, together with many other adaptive mechanisms which have helped the human race survive over the years.

Thus the things that we think of as normal values and attributes continue from generation to generation, because they adapt us for our environment and ensure the survival of our species.

Summary of Sections 1 and 2

- To be 'well adapted' is to be fit for a particular purpose.

- The human female body is well adapted for child bearing.

- Babies are well adapted for survival and for a long period of dependence.

- We can observe many features which have survival value in people who are in difficult or life-threatening situations.

- The things which we think of as 'normal' are those which have helped humans to survive in the past.

3: Natural selection

The way in which this process of adaptation has taken place has always been the subject of controversy, because it begins to impinge on matters of religious belief. This lies outside the scope of this unit. Here I am going to present a view which is widely accepted by geneticists and other scientists at the present time.

There is a lot of evidence to show that in plants, animals and micro-organisms some attributes are favoured over the course of time through a natural process.

This is termed **natural selection**. It results in those creatures who have attributes favourable to survival living to reproductive age, and therefore passing on their DNA to the next generation. The genes controlling those attributes are passed on, while the less favourable genes gradually become less and less frequent. This is what we see in the development of antibiotic resistant strains of bacteria in hospital.

In a hospital ward, there are many bacteria of different kinds. The **staphylococci** – 'staphs' – form a large group, some of which cause wound infections and other problems. In the past, most staphs were destroyed by antibiotics. In any particular hospital, nearly all the staphs (the whole population in that place) would be susceptible to the concentrations of antibiotics used in clinical practice. However, it seems that a few individuals in each population were resistant to these concentrations of antibiotics. When all the others were killed off, the resistant bacteria were free to grow and multiply rapidly, as there was no competition from the normal staphs. So in time, the whole population came to consist of resistant staphs. Unfortunately, these bacteria are capable of developing multiple resistance if single antibiotics are used in a concentration which does not kill them all off.

This is why it is emphasised to patients that they should always complete a course of prescribed antibiotics. *Methicillin resistant staphyloccus aureus* (MRSA) is a serious problem in hospitals.

Most geneticists believe that a similar process has taken place in the human species up to the present day – although there is a lot of debate about how it happened.

Before we began to control our environment, human beings were adapted in different ways to survive in different parts of the world. It is only in comparatively recent times that we have started moving around and exposing ourselves to conditions for which we are not well adapted. In the next section, we will look at an example of what happens under these circumstances.

4: A nice healthy tan?

Skin colour is a varying characteristic which you might have noted in *Activity 4*. In general, the darker skin tones are found in the areas of the world where people are exposed to strong sunlight. The skin pigment protects them from the damaging rays of the sun.

People who live in northern Europe are genetically rather varied because of all the waves of invasion and retreat which have taken place in the past. So in these regions, there is a wide range of skin tone. However, many people retain the pale, freckled skin and auburn hair of their distant ancestors, who lived for many generations under overcast skies. These people had no need for protective pigmentation, so their descendants are not well adapted for prolonged exposure to strong sunshine.

Now that travel has become easier and cheaper, an attractive suntan has become very desirable for pale-skinned northerners. As a result, many of them change their environment and spend parts of the year in the sun. Since they lack protection, they are at risk from skin damage.

The most serious damage is the production of skin cancer. **Malignant melanoma** is a very invasive cancer which originates in the pigmented cells of the skin. Its incidence has increased dramatically in recent years, both in Britain and, to a greater degree, in Australia. It is most common in people who have fair, freckled skin and is believed to be directly caused by sudden exposure to the harmful rays of the sun.

This condition is produced when people move into an environment for which they are not well adapted. It is an example of how **maladaptation** can lead to ill health.

5: One step ahead?

Humans have succeeded in moving into nearly all environments on the earth. Technological advances have enabled us to live comfortably in places for which we are not well adapted. Here is an example of the way that genetics is helpful in the process of preventing the adverse effects of changing our environment.

ACTIVITY 38   ALLOW **15** MINUTES

People who are at risk of malignant melanoma are now given plenty of health education advice. However, there is a short-term problem for people who have already had a lot of exposure to strong sunlight.

Read *Resource 6* – a short report of a new approach to this problem.

Then write one or two sentences describing what these researchers are attempting to do.

Commentary

You might have written a sentence like this:

The researchers are using a protein absent from melanoma cells to stimulate the immune system to attack the cancer cells.

If this approach is successful, natural selection for the protective genes will no longer take place and, in time, the genetic make-up of the human race will be slightly changed.

This example is only one of many ways in which modern medicine is setting aside the process of natural selection in human beings. Some say that natural selection no longer operates, since we have overcome nature and the environment. Other people say that it now works on a different basis. We have changed our environment and now present our genes with a new set of challenges.

Could it be that the people who survive to reproduce in the future will be those who are genetically adapted to resist the environmental challenges of modern life? There are no answers to this question yet, but the next activity should provide you with some food for thought on this topic.

ACTIVITY 39   ALLOW 20 MINUTES

Resource 7 deals with one of the environmental hazards we all have to face – atmospheric pollution from motor vehicles. It gives a comprehensive account of the threats to health which arise from this source.

Read the article carefully. Assuming that the structure and function of the lungs is under genetic control, what sort of genes are likely to help people to survive in heavily polluted environments? For example, the article starts with a description of how foreign particles are removed from the lungs.

You might well decide that a survival advantage would be conferred by any genes which were responsible for strong ciliary action in the upper respiratory tract. You could call this the 'strong cilia' gene.

Make a list of other similar survival genes. You may decide to do this alone, or you could work with a group of colleagues.

Commentary

Apart from the 'strong cilia' gene I have already mentioned, you could have listed genes for:

- abundant nasal hair
- active macrophages
- unrestricted airways
- strong coughing reflex
- mucal protection from sulphur dioxide and nitrogen dioxide
- abundant sulphite oxidase.

In doing this, you are building a genetic model for adaptation to a modern industrial environment.

It should be clear from your work on *Activity 39* that if people were exposed to this kind of environment for many generations those with the genes on your list would be able to function better than those without. They would tend to have more surviving children.

We would say that, under these conditions, that particular set of people were more **biologically fit** than others. The adaptive characteristics which they possessed would, over the course of time, become 'normal' characteristics and they would persist as long as the environmental conditions remained the same.

Summary of Sections 3 to 5

Characteristics that contribute to human survival have been favoured by natural selection.

- This is the process through which animals who are well adapted survive into their reproductive years and pass on their favourable genes to their offspring.

- Skin pigmentation is an adaptive feature, conferring protection against strong sunshine.

- Malignant melanoma has become more common as people without this adaptation expose themselves to excessive sunshine.

- Medical and technological advances are sometimes designed to allow us to avoid the consequences of maladaptation.

- In many ways, our activities appear to be modifying the course of natural selection in human beings.

I have provided you with an explanation of the way that the genes which govern our 'normal' characteristics come to be selected. However, we know that there are also many unfavourable genes. We might ask, 'How is it that these genes do not die out in the natural course of things?'.

There are two possible explanations. The first is that these unfavourable genes keep cropping up at random by means of a genetic change. I will deal with this at some length in the final section.

The second explanation is that, although the genes have some unfavourable effects, they also confer some adaptive benefits. This explanation is consistent with the idea that genes and their products do not exist in isolation from one another. There is one well-documented example which illustrates how this happens.

6: The paradox of sickle cell disease

In the case study of the child Karima – which you looked at on page 20 – I described a condition which is caused by a change in one of the genes responsible for the production of adult Hb. This change resulted in a failure to produce part of the Hb molecule. Many other small changes can take place in this gene. Some of them are like thalassaemia, and stop Hb production altogether. Others produce altered Hb.

The change occurring in **sickle cell disease** is of this kind.

The faulty gene is called Hb(S). It produces Hb with a slightly altered sequence of amino acids, which results in a change in its oxygen-carrying properties. When oxygen is in short supply, this altered Hb collapses and causes the red blood cells to become distorted – they become sickle-shaped. They then tend to stick in small blood vessels, blocking them and cutting off the blood supply, and so leading to tissue damage, infection and painful feverish episodes. The outcome is often fatal.

This disease is very widespread in African countries south of the Sahara desert, and is a serious health problem for many people of African descent.

But if the Hb(S) gene produces such serious effects, why does it persist in these populations? In the next activity, you will consider some of the evidence about this gene and see if you can answer this question.

ACTIVITY 40 — ALLOW 10 MINUTES

Here are a number of statements about sickle cell anaemia. Using them all, together with some of the knowledge you have already gained in this unit, write a brief answer to the question:

Why does the Hb(S) gene persist in the African population?

1   This gene exists in two alternative forms, the normal and the sickle. We call them Hb and Hb(S) respectively.
2   People who have two Hb(S) copies of the gene are affected by the illness.
3   People with two normal Hb or one normal plus one Hb(S) gene are not affected.
4   The spread of this disease is very similar to the distribution of malaria in Africa.
5   People with two normal Hb genes are more easily affected by the malarial parasite – which gets into red blood cells – than people with one Hb(S) gene.

Use the space below for your answer.

Commentary

The items of information above suggest that the Hb(S) gene persists because it confers some protection from the malarial parasite. If people with one Hb(S) gene are more resistant to malaria, they will tend to survive better in malarial regions and keep the faulty gene circulating in the population.

This example shows how a gene can have a number of different effects, and its persistence will depend on the environmental factors which affect its survival. So the way that genes are selected is rather more complex than it may have seemed at first sight.

7: Adaptation in patients and clients

It could be said that a person who is well adapted to a particular environment is in a state of 'health'. As far as our patients and clients are concerned, it is important to be aware of the extent to which they are genetically adapted to a particular situation and to help them to make the maximum use of what they have. Let's go back to one of our case studies and see how this idea applies.

ACTIVITY 41   ALLOW 5 MINUTES

Here is some additional information to add to our case study of Pauline, the older of the two women with breast cancer described on page 36.

As you read it through, think about her past and present life situation. Can you identify any adaptive or maladaptive features? Do you consider Pauline to be 'biologically fit'? Note down your response in the space that follows the activity.

Pauline's case study

Pauline was married at the age of 19 in 1929. She had five children, born between 1930 and 1944. They all survived the usual childhood illnesses and now all have families of their own. Pauline now has twenty grandchildren and two great-grandchildren.

Her husband was killed in action at the end of the Second World War. She worked to support her family in a heavy industrial job during and after the war, and continued to work in a series of domestic and catering jobs until she was 65.

Although she has never been well off and has suffered several serious illnesses, she rarely complains and tends to put up with things rather than make a fuss. She is a heavy smoker and says that she always has been.

Pauline detests being in hospital. She remains stoical but is very frightened and uncomfortable in these surroundings. She doesn't say much to the doctors and nurses, and tends to nod in agreement when they speak to her about her condition. Privately, she tells her daughters that she 'can't make head nor tail of what they say', and that she feels very embarrassed about her breast lesion and the symptoms which go along with it.

Commentary

It could be said that Pauline is very biologically fit, as she has a large number of surviving descendants. Her children were born during times of difficulty and hardship. She is clearly a 'hardy' person and must have been well adapted for her own life circumstances.

Her smoking could be seen as a maladaptive feature. However, some people might say that as it hasn't done her any harm, it could have helped her through difficult times. This is a debatable point which you might like to discuss with your colleagues.

She doesn't seem to be well adapted to her present situation in hospital. This is where the health-care staff can help her either to return to her familiar surroundings where she is comfortable or to build on her strength and independence in order to help her adapt to the necessary time in hospital.

ACTIVITY 42   ALLOW 30 MINUTES

Some writers on nursing have used the idea of adaptation as the basis of nursing theory. You might like to conclude this section by reading from the works of Callista Roy to see how her model fits in with the ideas on adaptation which we derive from our study of genetics (see Further Reading).

Summary of Sections 6 and 7

- Genes which confer a survival advantage persist and give rise to 'normal' characteristics.

- 'Unfavourable' genes can arise by random mutation.

- 'Unfavourable' genes may persist because they also confer some adaptive advantage.

- Health-care personnel have an important role to play in enabling patients and clients to adapt to a particular health situation.

You have now reached the end of Session Three. Before you move on to Session Four, check that you have achieved the objectives given at the beginning of this session, and, if not, review the appropriate sections.

SESSION FOUR

Vulnerability

Overview

In the first three sessions of this unit, I have described how – as a result of random genetic processes – the human body has come to be so beautifully adapted for life on this planet.

We have just touched on the intricacies of the genetic code.

During these discussions, I have mentioned 'faulty' genes and referred to conditions in which something goes seriously wrong with the genetic instructions – as in thalassaemia, haemophilia, melanoma and breast cancer. Understanding how things can go wrong, what makes them go wrong and why, is the area covered by our final key concept – the vulnerability of the genetic material.

Session objectives

When you have completed this session you should be able to:

- summarise the causes of genetic variation
- suggest how the environment can cause genetic damage
- explain the links between random changes and ageing
- outline how genetic repair mechanisms work
- give examples of new developments in gene therapy
- apply these principles to patient care.

Please note this text is written so that it can be understood by people who have not studied genetics at all in the past. It may be you have already achieved these outcomes and wish to use the material for revision purposes.

1: Variation and mutation

We begin this section by looking at yet another genetic cause of variation. We have already seen that 'normal' genes can exist in several alternative forms and that 'faulty' genes occur from time to time. Changes and mistakes in the genetic code obviously occur. But how and why does this happen?

This is the question which we are now going to explore.

Mutation

A change in a gene is known as a mutation. It results from a change in the sequence of letters in the genetic instruction. So the deliberate mistake which you made in *Activity 8* represented a mutation.

ACTIVITY 43   ALLOW 3 MINUTES

Refer back to *Activity 8* – on page 19 – and remind yourself of the three ways in which a single letter in the genetic instructions could be changed.

1

2

3

Commentary

In *Activity 8* you either:

- removed a letter
- added a letter

or

- substituted a letter.

These are the three ways in which a real-life single-letter mutation can occur.

However, mutations can also involve larger pieces of the code. A whole sentence can be deleted or made unreadable. So let's consider what brings this about, and why the genetic material is vulnerable to changes of this kind.

The causes of mutation

When cells anywhere in the body divide, the DNA in the nucleus is copied exactly. We have seen that the DNA is a very long strand, and you may already have wondered how something like this could possibly be copied.

Without going into the details of DNA structure, it is difficult to describe this process unless we use another metaphor.

Imagine this time that the DNA is like a very long zip fastener. In order to make an exact copy, it must be unzipped and a new half built on to each of the separated halves. Perhaps you could form a mental picture of the zip being undone from one end and, as the two halves come apart, new teeth are put in place so that two new zips grow from the original.

As the new 'zips' grow, mistakes can happen. Pieces can be missed out, or the wrong ones put in. Very roughly, this is what happens when a mutation occurs.

The DNA is vulnerable to these mistakes because it undergoes this copying process whenever a cell divides. Each time copying occurs, there is an opportunity for mistakes to happen. It appears that very often, the mutation occurs without apparent cause. It is a spontaneous mutation, due to the random movement of molecules at the time of cell division. At other times, a mutation may be associated with particular circumstances such as the presence of chemicals or some kinds of radiation. In this case, the mutation is assumed to have been caused by this environmental feature.

The factor that causes a mutation is called a **mutagenic agent**.

2: Mutagenic agents

Sometimes the press carries alarming stories about the mutagenic properties of common substances such as caffeine in coffee. Almost any chemical substance can cause mutations if it gets to the DNA in sufficient strength, but the reality is that the nucleus is protected from most harmful substances for most of the time by the body's own chemistry. It is very difficult to say which substances in what concentrations cause mutations in humans because, of course, we can't perform the necessary experiments.

However, it is possible to test chemicals for their potential to cause mutations in bacteria and it has been found that nearly all of those which cause mutations can also be shown to cause animal cancers. So the link between mutation and cancer is strong, as we will see later.

Radiation of various kinds is also linked to mutations and to cancers. If the energy in the radiation reaches the nucleus it can knock out parts of the nuclear material. Radiation arises from many sources, including the rocks of the earth itself – some of which contain radon, a radioactive gas. In health care, X-rays are a type of radiation which we commonly encounter. There is a particular concern about the cumulative effects of X-rays on the dividing cells in the sex organs, and so patients and carers are protected by lead shields when X-rays are being used for diagnostic or therapeutic purposes.

Although the link between radiation and mutation has been clearly shown by laboratory work, it is not clear just how much radiation exposure will cause genetic damage. Where people are frequently exposed to radiation, as in hospital X-ray departments, their exposure is carefully monitored and very cautious standards are set.

The next activity focuses on the difficulty of describing the exact effect of radiation on people.

ACTIVITY 44   ALLOW 10 MINUTES

The link between leukaemia and radiation exposure is strong.

Take a few minutes to read *Resource 8*, which deals with the arguments for and against the relationship between nuclear power stations and clusters of leukaemia cases. Then answer the following questions.

1 What is the latest theory, quoted in the article, about the link between leukaemia and lymphoma and radiation?

2 According to this theory, which tissues are most at risk from radiation?

Commentary

The author of the article in *Resource 8* points out that none of the evidence is conclusive. However, he describes a recent study which links these diseases in young people to their father's work in the nuclear industry. According to this theory, damage to the testes would cause defects in the sperm, which leads to leukaemia later in the next generation.

Summary of Sections 1 and 2

- A mutation is a change in the sequence of sub-units in the DNA of a gene.

- Mutations can occur during the replication of DNA. The genetic material is especially vulnerable at this time.

- Mutations also result from the influence of mutagenic agents.

- Radiation is a cause of genetic damage. Dividing tissues are especially vulnerable.

3: The results of mutation

Whether a mutation is spontaneous or caused by a mutagen, the result is almost always detrimental. This is because, over the long history of the human race, most mutations that can happen have happened and have been 'tried out' through the process of natural selection. The forms of the genes which now exist in the human genome are the best for our present purpose, so they are the ones that have survived.

Mutations can occur in any cells of the body. If a mutation occurs somewhere other than the sex organs, its effects will be confined to the person in whom it occurs. However, if the mutation happens where eggs or sperm are being formed, it may affect the chromosomes which are passed on to the next generation and its effects will be seen in the children, as described in *Resource 8*, or possibly in later generations if this mutation produces a recessive gene. This is what is thought to have happened in the case of Queen Victoria's family.

ACTIVITY 45	ALLOW **10** MINUTES

Look back at Queen Victoria's family tree on page 9.

From this, you will see that two of her daughters were carriers of haemophilia and one of her sons was affected by the disease. Her father was not affected and there was no history of haemophilia in her mother's family.

Using this information, can you work out why we think the mutation happened in one of Queen Victoria's parents? Note down your ideas below.

Commentary

There are two possible explanations for the condition of Queen Victoria's children. Clearly, three of them received a faulty X chromosome from their mother. This could have been the result of three new mutations of the same kind in the Queen's ovaries, during the development of the eggs which were to form these three babies.

The second possibility is that a new mutation in the previous generation resulted in Queen Victoria herself having a faulty X chromosome, and thus being a carrier. This would mean that half her eggs would be carriers and half her sons affected.

Of these two explanations, the second is most likely. A single mutation in one of Queen Victoria's parents is much more likely than three new mutations of the same kind in the Queen herself. However, in the field of random events, 'unlikely' is not the same as 'impossible'! So the first explanation cannot be ruled out entirely.

What about the ratio of affected to unaffected children in Queen Victoria's family? If the second explanation is true, we would expect half her sons to be affected and half her daughters to be carriers.

ACTIVITY 46   ALLOW 3 MINUTES

Check out the family tree on page 9 again and see if this is the case.

Suggest an explanation for what you observe, assuming that our second explanation is true.

Commentary

The Queen had five daughters, two of whom were carriers. This is close to half her female offspring. She had four sons, but only one was affected by haemophilia.

Although this is just one quarter of her male children, it could be the result of chance – or she might have had more male conceptions which, because of this defect, were spontaneously aborted. We can't choose between these possibilities, but the evidence we do have still supports the second explanation.

You will have noticed that we said the mutation could have happened in either of the Queen's parents. We do not know which one, because each parent transmitted an X chromosome to their daughter and there is no way of knowing which of these was faulty.

It is most likely that, either by chance or influenced by some environmental factor, this mutation took place in the actively dividing tissues of a royal ovary or testis. This is a very graphic example of the effects of the vulnerability of genetic material, and the consequences of a mutation in the sex organs. It highlights the need for protection of these organs from mutagenic agents, such as radiation.

When a mutation like this occurs, its effects are not likely to last for many generations. Exceptionally, an unfavourable mutation will confer some other advantage and will therefore persist, as in the case of the sickle cell gene.

It follows from this that some mutations must keep on occurring because, even though they reduce biological fitness, we find their effects in every generation.

They are most unlikely to be passed on from one generation to the next, so they must be happening anew from time to time. The next section considers what is known about their rate of occurrence.

4: How frequent are mutations?

Some genetic defects can be traced back into history for a long time. For example, we have already seen that classical haemophilia was present in the British and European royal families during the last century. But it was also recognised more than 2,000 years ago, and is mentioned in the Talmud, where regulations concerning circumcision make special allowance for boys in families where a 'bleeding' disease exists. So genes like this must arise continually, although rarely.

It is estimated from population studies that the haemophilia mutation occurs spontaneously about 40 times in every million eggs and sperms in each generation. Similar calculations have been made for a number of genetically determined illnesses, such as Duchenne muscular dystrophy, all of which show a low but constant rate of new mutations.

There are, however, many mutations which do not result in dramatic effects but which, together, cause a gradual accumulation of wear and tear. Such accumulated 'mistakes' are involved in the ageing process, which we will return to at the end of this unit. First, we need to consider the mutations which give rise to a very high proportion of human illness – those associated with malignant tumours.

Summary of Sections 3 and 4

- Most mutations are detrimental.
- A mutation in the sex cells will be passed on to the next generation.
- Mutations occur at a low but constant rate.

5: The genetics of tumour production

Benign tumours

It is very common for groups of cells somewhere in the body to grow more than they should and form a lump or bump of some sort. These cells have been changed in some way – perhaps by a viral mutagen – and they increase in number but do not spread to other parts of the body.

These are **benign** tumours, such as warts and many kinds of breast lumps. They may be a nuisance, and even dangerous if they cause pressure on a vital organ by their size, but in most cases they do not present a serious problem. However, it is vital to distinguish them from invasive tumours.

Malignant tumours

Cancers are **malignant** tumours. They consist of cells in which the processes of growth and differentiation have gone out of control. After an initial period of growth, the primary cancer invades adjacent tissues and spreads to other parts of the body, setting up secondary cancers – **metastases**. The cells of the cancer become increasingly abnormal and their chromosomes show many changes. Clearly, something has gone seriously wrong with their genetic information.

There are over 200 different types of human cancers, all having different characteristics. They are classified according to the tissue in which they arise.

So leukaemias are cancers of the white blood cells, and carcinomas are cancers of the covering and lining tissues of the body – the epithelial tissues. Although there is such a vast range of different cancers, there are some things which we can say in general terms about them.

1   Malignant tumours arise from mutations in single cells.

Usually these are somatic cells – cells which are not part of the egg- and sperm-forming tissues. So the effects of the mutations are confined to the person in whom the cancer arises and are not passed on to the next generation.

However, there are a few cancers which seem to be inherited in a clear-cut pattern or to show a family tendency. These result from mutations in the parent's sex cells which produce defects in their children's genetic material. Such defects have a knock-on effect as they increase the risk of cancerous changes in the offspring. Most of these cancers show up in the early years of life, when the most active cellular growth is taking place.

2   Malignant tumours show uncontrolled growth.

Normal cells respect the boundaries between themselves and adjacent tissues. They remain attached in the place where they should be, and their growth is regulated when the tissue which they make up reaches its appropriate size. Cancer cells appear to escape from this control, lose their attachments to their neighbours and thus spread through the body.

3   Regulator genes are involved in the development of cancers.

Although the reasons for these changes are not yet understood, it is clear that they result from changes in the genes which regulate the way that the cell divides and grows. In some cancers, it is now possible to identify specific regulator genes which are abnormal. These are called **oncogenes**. The name means 'tumour producing', but it is important to stress that these genes are not there to 'produce cancer'.

They normally do something else, but when they undergo a mutation they become involved in tumour production. Some of these oncogenes are normally involved with the production of the proteins which give the signals for cells to divide or which enable cells in a tissue to stick together. Defects in these mechanisms will clearly change the rate of cell division and interfere with the proper position of tissue cells.

When oncogenes are activated in the tissues from which the blood cells are formed, uncontrolled production of abnormal white cells occurs. All these white cells leave no room for production of red blood cells and platelets, which are involved in blood clotting. This gives rise to the anaemia and bruising which are characteristics of acute or chronic leukaemia.

4   Cancers are often induced by specific environmental factors.

The leukaemias, for example, are often shown to be associated with exposure to radiation. The next activity looks at these environmental factors.

ACTIVITY 47   ALLOW 5 MINUTES

There are lots of varying ideas about what causes cancers and what one needs to avoid in order to minimise the risk. No doubt you have heard or read about several things which are suspected of causing different cancers. Some of them have been mentioned already in this unit – for example, ultraviolet light as a cause of skin cancers.

Make a list of the environmental causes that you have heard or read about.

Commentary

So far in this unit I have discussed:

- ● ultraviolet light as a cause of skin cancer
- ● other types of radiation as a cause of leukaemia
and
- ● various chemical substances as causes of unspecified cancers.

You may have listed various other things, including:

- ● cigarette smoke, which contains over 50 carcinogenic substances
- ● dietary factors
- ● viruses
- ● industrial chemicals.

The list of potential cancer-causing agents – **carcinogens** – is very long and makes depressing reading. It seems as if environmental hazards are all around us.

This is certainly true, but the picture is not as gloomy as it first appears. In the case of all these carcinogens, it is quite clear that not everyone who is exposed to them develops cancer. It seems that we have some inbuilt protective mechanisms.

6: Now for the good news

The more we learn about the genetic information in cell nuclei, the more we come to appreciate its sophistication. So far in this section, we have been describing the vulnerability of DNA, particularly at the time when copies are being made.

However, new findings in genetics are gradually revealing that the genetic material contains its own self-correcting systems.

Picking up our earlier metaphor of a book, we could say that the DNA instruction manual not only writes itself but also does its own proof-reading and correction!

This happens in two ways:

- Firstly, as the DNA is being copied and the new strands are forming from the original, any 'letter' which is incorrectly placed will be removed by a part of the cellular machinery. This checking process deals with most of the mistakes which occur by deletion, addition or omission of a letter in the code sequence. Only a few are overlooked, and so spontaneous mutations occur at the low frequencies which we described earlier.

- Secondly, it is known that some of the damage produced by carcinogenic agents can be repaired. If the DNA is damaged by agents such as ultraviolet light, there are parts of the cellular machinery that can snip out the defective region and fill in the gap that is created.

In these and other similar ways the genetic material is protected. Some cancerous conditions are caused by a failure of these protective mechanisms. Overall they explain why our genetic material is often capable of withstanding severe environmental hazards.

This is not to say that these hazards should be disregarded. Because there are people around who have smoked twenty cigarettes a day all their life and live to be over eighty (like Pauline in our case study) it would be unwise for most of us to ignore the risks associated with smoking. We cannot say which people are the most vulnerable. But it is helpful to take a balanced view of the many environmental risks we face and the response of our cells to these risks.

7: More good news

This particular unit is being written at a time when advances in genetic science are occurring at an astonishing rate. It sometimes seems that every day we read about promising new lines of treatment for specific cancers and for other illnesses caused by faulty genes, such as certain cardiovascular diseases.

Geneticists are looking forward to a time, about ten to twenty years from now, when it should be possible to detect the gene for inherited early-onset breast cancer within a young woman's body cells and thus identify those who are genetically at risk.

These developments provide us with much encouragement but also raise difficult questions about what can and should be done as a result of this increasing knowledge.

*over the course
of a week*

ACTIVITY 48

ALLOW **60** MINUTES

We have put together a compilation of some recent press articles on advances in genetic therapy. You will find these compiled under the title

'Activity 48', as *Resource 9*. Of course, knowledge is developing so fast that by the time you read this unit, things may have changed!

Over the course of about a week, review the papers and your professional journals to see how often these topics are mentioned. Compare your findings with the compilation in *Resource 9*, which dates from December 1992. You will probably need to make notes on a separate sheet, but you could summarise these below.

Now let's take stock before continuing with the session.

Summary of Sections 5 to 7

- Tumours often arise as a result of mutation.

- Malignant tumours exhibit uncontrolled growth.

- Oncogenes are involved in the regulation of cell growth. If these become faulty, malignant tumours may result.

- Some cancers are associated with specific environmental factors.

- The nucleus contains its own 'repair mechanisms' which counter the effects of mutations.

- The development of knowledge concerning the genetics of cancer is one of the most rapidly expanding areas of science at present.

8: Understanding ageing

As people grow older, their characteristics change. It is popularly supposed that this is simply a 'wearing-out' process. However, some of the new advances in genetics seem to point towards the view that ageing is programmed into our genetic composition and that, before too long, it may be possible to predict a person's natural lifespan. Perhaps we might look at ageing more closely from a biological perspective.

As we emphasised in the previous section, the human body is adapted to produce and nurture dependent offspring. If this process continued over a longer period of adult life, there would soon be far too many people for comfort. So we might say that it is in the interests of the human species as a whole that each of us eventually gives way to the next generation. In other words, ageing is an adaptive process.

ACTIVITY 49   ALLOW 5 MINUTES

In Session One, when you looked for characteristics which run in families, did you notice any that were to do with the length of life? Think back to that family again and see if you can detect any characteristics of this kind.

Commentary

It is not uncommon to find families with long-lived, active members in successive generations. Of course, it could be that this reflects environmental factors, but it might also suggest a genetic tendency to age at a slower rate than most people. In our case study, Pauline's family is just such an example. Her mother lived to be over 90 and did her own housework up to the day she died. Pauline has two older sisters and a brother alive today, all over 85. They, like Pauline, remain lively and active.

One way that ageing occurs is by the accumulation of random mistakes in the genetic material over a lifetime. As we explained earlier, many of these are corrected, but some persist, and will gradually begin to cause problems. Most very elderly people have a number of slow-growing tumours.

We also know that genes are switched on at different times in our lives. Some of the illnesses of old age are known to arise from a genetic defect which does not appear until middle age at the earliest. There are likely to be other genetic causes of ageing and of the rate at which it takes place. So it may be that, for each of us, our genetic book of instructions not only writes and corrects itself as it goes along, but has already written its ending.

The more we come to understand human genetics, the closer we come to being able to read the ending. This sort of information will have a profound influence on the future of health care. For a few conditions associated with ageing, that future is here and now, as the next activity demonstrates.

ACTIVITY 50   ALLOW 15 MINUTES

Resource 10 is an article written by a nurse specialist in genetics. It deals with **Alzheimer's disease,** which is a common condition causing dementia in elderly people. Some cases of Alzheimer's begin much earlier, and this type is especially common in people with Down syndrome which, as you will recall, is a chromosomal abnormality caused by an extra small chromosome.

In this article, the author is discussing some families in which early-onset Alzheimer's has a genetic cause. It is important to stress that most cases of this condition seem to arise from other causes and are not necessarily inherited.

With this information in mind, read *Resource 10*, concentrating on the role of the nurse specialist in working with families where there is a clear genetic cause. When you have finished, try to answer the following questions.

1 What important functions does the nurse have in working with families which carry the burden of genetic disease?

2 What, in your opinion, is the greatest challenge for health carers who are supporting the younger members of families with inherited Alzheimer's?

Commentary

The article describes several aspects of this specialist nursing function, including:

- contacting family members
- giving information
- assessing their need for support
- clarifying misconceptions
- taking pedigrees (family trees)
- liaison with other professionals
- dealing with the emotional responses of family members as the disease progresses.

The author describes a situation in which it is possible to detect the gene responsible for this fatal degenerative disease. Health carers here are dealing with people who know that they have a one-in-two chance of developing the illness which is unfolding in their parent. It is possible for those people to take a blood test and then to be almost sure if they will or will not become ill. This is clearly a terrible situation for them, especially if they already have children of their own. It represents an enormous challenge for health carers both in supporting the younger family members, assisting them to make informed choices and dealing with the consequences of taking the test, if that is what they choose.

There is a great deal more to be said about ageing and about the role of health carers in working with ageing people. In this section, I have approached this subject from the angle of the vulnerability of the genetic material and have tried to show that there is more to the process than just wearing out. Rather, ageing is part of our natural life cycle, whether it occurs early in the context of illness or at the end of a long lifespan.

Before concluding this unit, let's take a final look at our two case studies, moving on six months from when we last encountered Mary and Pauline.

ACTIVITY 51   ALLOW **10** MINUTES

First, read the next instalment of our two case studies.

An update on Pauline

Pauline has now been discharged from hospital. She has returned to her own home and attends an oncology unit twice a week on a day basis, where she has her ulcer dressed and joins in with a range of social activities. She has had a course of radiotherapy to the ulcer which has reduced its size and made it less distressing. She is looking forward to a large family party with her brother, sisters and all the children and grandchildren at Christmas.

An update on Mary

Mary has also had radiotherapy. She felt very unwell during the process but now her symptoms have improved and she too has gone home. She is very frail but is determined to see Christmas and share it with her children. She realises that it may be her last.

Before leaving the hospital, she talked at length with a member of staff about her fears for her daughter's future. She is very concerned that the child may also be at risk from inherited early-onset breast cancer.

You now have all the available information about Pauline and Mary. I suggest that you now review the whole of their case studies, on pages 36, 37, 66, 67, 79, 80 and 94.

When you have completed your review, think about the ideas relating to genetic vulnerability which we have been discussing in this section. Consider what the case studies tell us about the vulnerability of these two women to genetic damage.

Commentary

There is a striking contrast between Mary and Pauline in terms of their vulnerability to genetic damage. Because Mary is one of the small proportion of breast cancer sufferers who are unfortunate enough to inherit the defective gene, the dice were loaded against her from the start. During her pregnancy, the environment in her body favoured the rapid development and spread of the cancer.

Pauline seems to have been much less vulnerable, surviving many environmental hazards and ageing slowly, like other members of her family. It looks as if she got dealt a good deal genetically.

Both women received radiotherapy to treat their cancers. I have described radiation as a cancer-causing agent, so it may seem strange that it is used to cure cancer too. It can be used in this way because the rapidly dividing cancer cells are very vulnerable to radiation and can be killed off if the radiation dose is precisely targeted at them. However, this also affects other parts of the body, particularly where cells are dividing, and causes side effects such as digestive upsets. This is why Mary, who required radiotherapy to internal structures, felt so unwell.

Finally, Pauline doesn't have to worry about passing on her illness to her daughters, but Mary does. No one can tell her how likely it is that her daughters will inherit the gene, but she can be told about the rapid advances in detection and treatment of the condition, and the expectation of progress before her daughter reaches puberty. She can be given that kind of good news.

Summary of Section 8

- Ageing may be considered to be an adaptive process.

- The accumulation of random mistakes contributes to the ageing process.

- The early onset of Alzheimer's disease has a genetic basis.

- People vary in their vulnerability to genetic change.

9: Back to the family tree

Let's leave this unit as we began, with a look at the family tree. Go back to the family trees you constructed in *Activity 1*. You should be able to understand them much better now, and to apply what you have learnt.

For example, looking back at the two family trees that we constructed for PKU and hair colour (*Figures 1* and *2*) we can see that the illness appears to be inherited in a clear-cut fashion, whilst the hair colour does not. The family members are either unaffected or affected by PKU – there are no apparent intermediates. But some have red hair, and others are reddish blond. So it seems likely that hair colour is governed by several genes, whereas PKU is likely to be caused by a single faulty gene.

It is apparent that true red hair seems to skip generations. It was present in my mother's generation and in my children's, but not in mine. It would be interesting to see what the pattern was in the past, but unfortunately there are no records. In cases like this, we just have to wait and see what the future brings.

It is likely that the genes for this particular hair colour will go on into future generations of my family, but it looks as if the PKU gene might have faded out from the genome. This is clearly an unfavourable mutation, which must have occurred somewhere in my grandparents' generation, or earlier. Without additional knowledge we couldn't say if this gene is sex-linked or not. Both the affected children were boys, but there were no girls in that family.

If you consider your family tree, you may well find yourself in the same situation. You come across an inherited factor and you haven't got enough information to explain it. You can find out more from the books in the Further Reading section if you want to follow up something of this kind.

Reading up about PKU, we find that it is not a sex-linked condition. Both boys and girls are affected, so the faulty gene is not on the sex chromosomes. It is a recessive condition, and therefore the gene only shows up if the normal gene is not present.

This means that the affected person must have two copies of the faulty gene. They must be homozygous for the PKU gene, having received one copy from the father and one from the mother. Both parents must be carriers. So both parents of these children must have had one copy of the faulty gene: they were heterozygous for the PKU gene.

The father of these children was heterozygous and it could be that my mother – his sister – was also heterozygous, and could have passed the faulty gene to me.

Perhaps it has not faded from our genome after all … if I had married a man who was also heterozygous, then our children would have been at risk from this illness. Fortunately, I did not, but this was purely by chance, as it were. There was no way of knowing, and it would have been a random piece of bad luck if we had both turned out to be heterozygous for this gene.

So this family tree illustrates all the four concepts in this unit.

- It demonstrates a few of the variations between members of the same family.

- It shows how random genetic events produce different mixes of genes and how random selection of partners influences the outcome.

- We can see that some members of this family were less well adapted than others, and did not survive to pass on their genes.

- Somewhere in a previous generation, mutations occurred in the vulnerable genetic material of two people, resulting in the presence of the PKU gene in the heterozygous state in both of them.

Once you start to draw family trees like this, you will find many things to interest you in families that you know well.

We hope that this unit has given you an insight into the fascination of genetics and the way it can help us understand ourselves and those we care for. Perhaps it will encourage you to read further around some of the topics we have introduced.

LEARNING REVIEW

Now that you have completed your work on this unit, you may like to assess your progress and understanding. You can do this by completing the following learning review, and comparing your answers with those that you gave before you started Session One.

	Not at all	Partly	Quite well	Very well

Session One
I can:
- explain the relevance of genetics to health-care practice ☐ ☐ ☐ ☐
- give a simple explanation of the way in which genetic and environmental factors give rise to observable differences between people ☐ ☐ ☐ ☐
- explain, in non-technical terms, the nature and origins of the genetic code ☐ ☐ ☐ ☐
- describe how the genetic code is organised into genes ☐ ☐ ☐ ☐
- give examples of the way in which the environment affects gene expression ☐ ☐ ☐ ☐
- apply these ideas to care planning. ☐ ☐ ☐ ☐

Session Two
I can:
- explain the random nature of the inheritance of gender ☐ ☐ ☐ ☐
- explain how an understanding of the role of randomness in cell division enables genetic outcomes to be predicted ☐ ☐ ☐ ☐
- outline the basis of single-factor inheritance patterns ☐ ☐ ☐ ☐
- explain how random events contribute to genetic variation ☐ ☐ ☐ ☐
- describe the contribution of genes and the environment to the establishment of a 'normal' state ☐ ☐ ☐ ☐
- apply the ideas in this session to care planning. ☐ ☐ ☐ ☐

Session Three
I can:
- explain the advantages for survival of 'normal' characteristics ☐ ☐ ☐ ☐
- give examples of survival behaviour and explain its genetic basis ☐ ☐ ☐ ☐

	Not at all	Partly	Quite well	Very well
outline the effects on health of moving between environments	☐	☐	☐	☐
make links between the concepts of adaptation and health	☐	☐	☐	☐
suggest why characteristics may persist despite being unfavourable	☐	☐	☐	☐
apply these ideas to health-care practice.	☐	☐	☐	☐

Session Four

I can:

	Not at all	Partly	Quite well	Very well
summarise the causes of genetic variation	☐	☐	☐	☐
suggest how the environment can cause genetic damage	☐	☐	☐	☐
explain the links between random changes and ageing	☐	☐	☐	☐
outline how genetic repair mechanisms work	☐	☐	☐	☐
give examples of new developments in gene therapy	☐	☐	☐	☐
apply these principles to patient care.	☐	☐	☐	☐

RESOURCES SECTION

Contents

RESOURCE I

*Simon LeVay,
'Beyond belief',
The Guardian,
9 October 1992*

Are homosexuals born and not made?

Among the many bizarre notions that Sigmund Freud inflicted on the world, his ideas about male homosexuality must take pride of place.

He asserted that all young boys have a strong sexual bond with their mothers, a bond they have to break in order to develop sexual feelings towards other women. If, on account of the mother's close-binding behaviour, the father's hostility, or other reasons, a boy breaks this bond as an adult he will seek sexual partners with whom he can re-enact this role – this time taking the mother's part. Although Freud did not write extensively on female sexuality, he seems to have envisaged a mirror-image process to account for it.

Besides lacking supporting evidence, Freud's theory has two unfortunate consequences: first, within a homophobic society, it placed an undeserved burden of guilt on the parents of gays and lesbians. Second, it led to the notion of the 'curability' of homosexuality, a notion with traumatic consequences for many gay men.

Recently, research in various disciplines has been converging on quite a different picture. Neurobiologists have defined the brain circuits responsible for sex behaviour, and have shown that the sexual differentiation of these circuits takes place pre-natally under the influence of sex hormones such as testosterone.

Geneticists have demonstrated a strong influence of heredity on sexual orientation in both men and women. Child psychologists have shown that adult homosexuality is to some extent predictable on the basis of childhood characteristics such as gender-nonconformity in play. In turn, these childhood characteristics are known from both human and animal studies to be strongly influenced by genetic or hormonal factors operating before birth.

Finally, cognitive scientists have shown that gay men and lesbian women differ from their straight counterparts in a variety of perceptual and behavioural traits – such as verbal skills, and right- or left-handedness – that are most easily explained in terms of differences in pre-natal brain development.

In my own research, published a year ago, I described structural differences between gay and straight men in the anterior hypothalamus, the brain region most centrally involved in the production of typical male sex behaviour. More recently, Laura Allen and Roger Borski at the University of California, Los Angeles, reported on a second brain difference, this time in the anterior commissure, a pathway connecting the left and right hemispheres of the cerebral cortex. This difference may be related to some of the cognitive differences between gay and straight men mentioned above.

This is not to say we understand what makes people straight or gay. We do not. But the evidence strongly suggests that the factors influencing sexual orientation operate during the normal process of sexual differentiation of the brain, which occurs largely before birth.

Further progress will require the identification of genes that influence sexual orientation. If such genes are found it will be possible to ask when, where and how they exert their effects.

As far as the interests of the gay and lesbian communities are concerned, this whole area of research has the potential for both positive and negative consequences. The benefits may include a better understanding of the innate differences between gay and straight people, a rejection of homophobia based on religious or moral arguments, and the extension of greater legal protection to gays and lesbians.

The latter is especially important in countries such as the US where the constitutional protection of groups hinges critically on the demonstration of the 'immutability' of membership in a group. Until now, such protection for gays and lesbians has been rejected by the US courts on the grounds that homosexuality is a 'chosen lifestyle' and hence not immutable.

On the negative side, the current work may reinforce, albeit irrationally, the notion of homosexuality as a defect that can and should be 'fixed', or even prevented by means of pre-natal testing and selective abortion. In this connection it should be stressed that science itself has no definition for what is normal, and what is abnormal. Science can only describe what is out there and attempt to explain how it got that way. The acceptance of homosexuality as something normal and desirable depends above all on the image that gays and lesbians themselves present to society.

As a gay man, I believe that I can contribute more to my community by the openness and pride with which I conduct my life than by any amount of laboratory research.

Simon LeVay is a British-born neurobiologist on the faculty of the Salk Institute, La Jolla, California, and the University of California, San Diego. He founded the Institute of Gay and Lesbian Education in West Hollywood.

Gene therapy hope in muscular dystrophy

RESOURCE 2

Vines G, 'Muscular dystrophy could soon succumb to gene therapy', New Scientist 1992, 133, 1814, 24; Nursing Standard, Volume 6/Number 30/1992

A therapy which should lead to a substantial improvement in the quality of life for boys with Duchenne muscular dystrophy could be as little as five years away, researchers say.

The gene which is responsible for the condition was discovered five years ago and is known to produce dystrophin, a protein which spans the outer membrane of muscle cells. Now scientists have transferred a mini version of the genes into mice with a similar disorder.

Although the mice were not cured, there were signs of substantial improvement.

Between 19 and 28 per cent of muscle in these mice shows signs of damage but in the transgenic ones only 3–5 per cent of muscle fibres had been damaged. Serum creatine kinase was also reduced but not to normal levels. Before the gene could be used in humans some form of vehicle must be found for it. Retroviruses have been suggested, but the complete dystrophin gene is too big to fit within one.

Wound healing under the microscope

RESOURCE 3

Arthur Johnson, Community Outlook, January 1987

Arthur Johnson kicks off our special quarterly series on wound care in the community with an in-depth look at the healing process. What helps wounds to heal, and what inhibits them?

The healing process involves a complex series of events, initiated by trauma, death of tissues, or pathogenic invasion. The processes are best described as proceeding through three discrete phases: the inflammatory phase, the proliferative phase and the remodelling or differentiation phase.

The inflammatory phase

Trauma disrupts the dermal capillaries and lymph vessels, causing bleeding, and the release of kinins, histamine, serotonin, and intracellular enzymes. The immediate response of the body to trauma is to control bleeding, and to prevent the entry of pathogens.

Within seconds after injury, vaso-constriction occurs. Damaged tissues and platelets release thrombokinase and thromboplastin, counteracting the action of heparin, and causing the conversion of prothrombin into thrombin. The latter precipitates fibrinogen to fibrin.

Shed platelets release serotonin and ADP (adenosine diphosphate), causing aggregation of platelets, forming a clot stabilised by the fibrin net. This normally lasts for about 5–10 minutes.

Intracellular enzymes break down norepinephrine, causing venules to dilate and increasing blood flow to the wound site. Complement C3a anaphylatoxins provoke the release of histamine from mast cells and basophils, increasing vascular permeability to plasma proteins, antibodies, complement factors, and electrolytes, causing leakage of transudate into interstitial space in tissues around the wound.

Interaction between the damaged tissues and serum releases Cyclic AMP and complement by-products C3 and C5. Such complexes have been shown to be chemotactic to neutrophils. Furthermore, a fragment of human C3 complement factor (C3e) provokes a release of polymorphonuclear leucocytes from the bone marrow.

This means that the numbers of leucocytes in the circulation are greatly increased and are attracted to the wound site by chemotactic agents. Within a short time after injury or pathogenic invasion, neutrophils are attracted to the site of injury, and then adhere to the vascular endothelium. By a process known as diapedesis the neutrophils migrate through the vascular wall via interendothelial junctions, into the injured or infected tissues, and are thus made available for phagocytosis.

The destruction of pathogens is greatly enhanced by opsonins which help neutrophils to recognise bacteria, and then to adhere to them.

Antibodies, such as the immunoglobins of the IgG class, and fragments of C3, ie C3a and C3b, act as opsonins. In humans, C3b receptors can be demonstrated on the surface of most neutrophils, enabling the neutrophil to recognise and bind to the bacteria.

After invagination, the neutrophil ingests the bacterium, enclosing it in a vacuole called a phagosome. Lysosomal granules migrate towards the phagosome, and the membranes of the granules and phagosome fuse. The granules then rupture, discharging alkaline phosphatase and lysosome and the hydrolases. A complex series of metabolic events then occur, ending in the destruction of bacteria and particles. Numbers of neutrophils begin to decline as the bacterial population is eradicated, and macrophages become the dominant cell type. Macrophages begin to secrete chemotactic factor, attracting more macrophages to the wound site.

The lysosomes of macrophages contain hydrolytic enzymes which digest organic debris, and thus debride the wound of damaged or necrotic tissues. Simultaneously, antibody-antigen complexes inactivate toxins. By about day four after injury the wound is cleared of bacteria, toxins, dead tissues and foreign particles, preparing the way for the repair process.

Proliferative phase

Macrophages release monokines which affect the healing process in a number of ways. Activated macrophages secrete a factor which is chemotactic to fibroblasts.

Secondly, macrophages activate a serum component which stimulates fibroblast division, thus stimulating the multiplication of fibroblasts in the fibrotic base of the wound.

Thirdly, prostaglandin E2, is produced which activates the biosynthesis of collagenase, and fourthly macrophage action stimulates the synthesis of collagen.

The main role of fibroblasts is the synthesis of collagen. However, they can develop into modified cells called myofibroblasts, which give wound tissues the ability to contract; and fibroclasts, which assist in the remodelling phase.

The secretion of chemotactic factor by macrophages attracts fibroblasts to the wound site, and after synthesising the macromolecules of the extracellular matrix or ground substance, begin to synthesise collagen. Macrophages also secrete angiogenesis factor which is chemotactic to angioblasts, stimulating capillary bud formation. Thus the microcirculation is renewed, allowing a better supply of nutrients to the wound site. The wound cavity or base of the would is filled gradually with granulation tissue, that is ground substance, collagen, and capillary loops.

Remodelling phase

During the remodelling phase, the original collagen gel is replaced by a process of lysis and resynthesis, into a disorganised mass of collagen fibres. This process is aided by the fibroclasts. Further lysis and resynthesis occurs and interdigitation with proteoglycans results in an organised optimal orientation of the collagen fibres.

Intermolecular cross-linking and dehydration of the fibres further strengthens the scar, achieving maximum strength in about three months, but never more than 80 per cent of the strength of intact skin.

Epithelialisation

Epithelialisation involves the migration of epidermal cells from the perimeter of the wound, across the wound surface. In a shallow wound, sources of new epidermis are available from hair follicles, sebaceous glands, and the ducts of sweat glands. In full-thickness wounds, however, a clean, healthy base of granulation tissue is necessary to enable migration of epidermal cells from the wound perimeter.

Mature tissue cells produce chemical messengers called chalones, which inhibit cell division, or mitosis. If the amount of chalone in the extracellular fluid falls below a critical level, for example, through the loss of exudate, the cells are no longer inhibited from dividing, and a burst of mitotic activity ensues. As the cells multiply in numbers, the amount of chalone rises, slowing down mitosis, until complete healing is achieved, and mitosis ceases.

Mitosis is most intense in the epidermis surrounding the perimeter to the wound, and most activity occurs in a 3-mm width of epidermis immediately adjacent to the wound, gradually falling off in activity for 5 mm. G.D. Winter[2] described a leap-frog mechanism, whereby cells above the basal cell elongate and crawl over one another, until they make contact with the dermis, and become static. New cells crawl over the forerunners and in their turn colonise a further stretch of dermis, and so extend the regenerating sheet of cells.

The average speed of epidermal regeneration is approximately $7\mu m$, or roughly one cell diameter per hour. Migrating epidermal cells secrete a specific enzyme, a collagenase, which separates the fibrin/platelet scab from underlying tissues, enabling the epidermal cells to migrate across the underlying granulation tissue. Moisture at the wound surface is particularly important. Drying of the wound surface forces the cells to burrow deeper, until a moist level is found.

Clearly, wound healing is complex, but can be helped by effective nursing and the use of modern materials.

What should the doctor or nurse do (or not do) to influence the rate and quality of healing? Without a doubt, they should consider the whole patient, not just the wound. The treatment of underlying disease should be considered. For example, poor capillary blood supply can often be improved by the use of Stromba. This aids the lysis of fibrin cuffs around capillaries, thus improving blood supply. Oedema can be reduced by diuretics, elevation, intermittent compression, and rest.

The psychological aspects of a 'smelly' chronic ulcer can be devastating, leading to acute depression, poor diet, and isolation from family and friends. Effective control of the smell can be achieved using Lyofoam C and Odex gels. Elimination of the smell has been shown to improve a patient's attitude to treatment.

Attention to nutrition is most important, but requires more consideration than I can give it here. Large wounds can produce large metabolic disturbances, leading to protein wastage and the inhibition of insulin secretion. It is essential, therefore, that metabolic disturbances are prevented, or quickly rectified by an adequate diet, supplemented by vitamins A and C. The latter are required for collagen synthesis and epithelialisation.

There is now a consensus of opinion that routine zinc supplements are useless unless the serum zinc levels are very low. On the other hand, excessive zinc can inhibit phagocytosis, and affects the cross-linking of collagen.

Clearly, it is important to seek the advice of a dietician early, and to monitor serum protein, serum zinc, blood glucose, and haemoglobin levels regularly. The micro-environment between the wound and dressing can also directly influence healing processes.

There is a large range of new primary dressings designed to aid natural healing. They include:
● Semi-permeable adhesive films – Opsite, Tegaderm, Opraflex, Bioclusive, Ioban 2, Transigen, Tegaderm Pouch Dressing.
● Hydrocolloids – Vigilon, Scherisorb sheet, Scherisob gel, Geliperm.
● Polysaccharide dextranomers – Bard Absorption Dressing, Debrisan beads and paste, Iodosorb, Sorbasan, Kaltostat.
● Polyurethane foams – Lyofoam, Synthaderm, Coraderm.

Each group of dressings can be used for specific purposes. Some primary dressings for example, Opsite, may promote the cleavage of C3 and C5 complement factors, thus attracting neutrophils and macrophages to the wound site. Occlusive dressings, such as Granuflex, produce an anaerobic wound environment which stimulates angiogenesis, aids the debridement process and reduces the secretion of inflammatory mediators, thus significantly reducing pain levels. Hydrogel sheets, for example, Scherisorb sheet, quickly rectify overgranulation, while Lyofoam promotes and maintains mitotic activity, because of its superior thermal insulation properties. A mixture of Varidase and KY jelly, covered by an occlusive dressing will quickly debride necrotic tissue, while infected wounds can be cleared of pathogens in a few days by the application of Debrisan paste compresses.

What are the general characteristics of modern primary dressings, and how do they influence healing? High humidity is maintained between the wound and the dressing, enabling cells to migrate unhindered. In chronic wounds, high humidity prevents the formation of a dry scab across the wound surface, and scar formation is minimal. The practice of exposing wounds to the air should, on this evidence alone, be discontinued.

Primary dressings remove excess wound exudate from the wound surface. Some dressings absorb the exudate and form a gel, others are hydrophilic, draw in the exudate, and pass the exudate on to secondary dressings. Removal of excess exudate prevents maceration, and rids the wound of metabolic waste products, toxins, and dead cells.

Until the advent of occlusive dressings, gaseous exchange through the dressing to the wound surface was thought to be important. However, the hypoxic environment under occlusive dressings was shown to stimulate angiogenesis, and to contribute to sustained pain relief. The supply of oxygen via the microcirculation would, therefore, appear to be the most important route of transmission. Blowing oxygen onto the wound surface has been shown to lower wound surface temperature significantly, and dry it. Both factors inhibit natural healing processes.

Biological processes such as mitosis and enzymatic activity are greatly affected by changes in temperature. A constant wound surface of 37°C is essential to promote and maintain these processes. A drop of only 2°C is enough to slow down mitosis significantly. It is important, therefore, that the wound site is kept warm. Remove the dressing immediately before inspection, and then redress it immediately. Removing dressings some time before a doctor's round should be discouraged.

Dressing wounds with substances such as honey, sugar, marmite, yoghurt, egg-white and egg-yolk should be questioned, now that a range of safe, sterile primary dressings is available. There is now ample evidence[6] of the dangers of using hypochlorites such as Eusol in open wounds, yet they continue to be used. Hypochlorites have been shown to cause irreversible damage to the micro-circulation, and to interfere with fibroblastic function and collagen synthesis. Furthermore they attack coliform organisms, and release endotoxins. The latter are absorbed, and can produce a range of side-effects, varying from mild uraemic toxaemia to acute renal failure. There are safe alternatives to hypochlorites.

Materials of the future

Intense research is now being carried out into every aspect of wound healing and management.

Fibronectin, a substance found in serum, has caused great interest recently. Fibronectin aids the migration of cells such as fibroblasts, by forming fibrils along which the cells migrate. This explains how cells can find their target sites with such unerring accuracy.

The application of topical fibronectin may speed up the healing process. When included in eye drops, fibronectin has been shown to speed up the healing of corneal ulcers.

Research into synthetic skin replacements looks promising. Replacement skin derived from bovine collagen, sharks' fins, and polymers are already at the early stages of development. Methods of epidermal tissue culture look particularly exciting for the treatment of burns. By culturing a small sample of epidermis from two young brothers, with 97 per cent burns, Howard Green and colleagues at Harvard Medical School were able to replace more than 80 per cent of the children's skin. Both children now have smooth, functioning skin.

Transdermal medication is already possible using dressings such as the hydrogels, while micro-encapsulation of cells will enable transplantation of Islets of Langerhans into diabetic patients without problems of rejection. The future looks very exciting, but only if attitudes begin to change, and we are prepared to question what we do to patients.

References

[1]Schumann, D. The nature of wound healing. AORN Journal, 1982: 35: 1068–1077.

[2]Winter, G.W. Healing of skin wounds and the influence of dressings on the repair process. In Harkiss, J.J., Ed., Surgical Dressings and Wound Healing, Symposium, Bradford, July 7–8 1979. Bradford University Press/Crosby Lockwood: 1971.

[3]Turner, T.D. The functional development of wound management products, Proceedings of conference on Medical Applications of Textiles, Leeds University, 1981.

[4]Materials for medicine, Scientific American, October 1968, 97–103.

[5]Johnson, A. Clinical Evaluation of Lyofoam C., Journal of Tissue Viability, 'Care' September 1986.

[6]Brennan, S., Leaper, D. 'Antiseptics and Wound Healing. British Journal of Surgery 1985; 72: 780–782.

Arthur Johnson is district infection control officer with Darlington health authority.

RESOURCE 4

Sarah Stacey, Good Housekeeping, November 1992, Vol. 142 (5) pp205-209

Find out your future health

The key to your future health may lie in your past – in the genes you were born with. Sarah Stacey shows how you can trace your family's health history.

Every week, experts at Great Ormond Street Hospital for Sick Children gather to review the latest referrals to the genetics department. In a room lined with medical textbooks, 12 doctors swig coffee while they scrutinise patients' records and agree on a course of action.

These are clinical geneticists, who deal with patients rather than simply doing research. Unusually among the medical establishment, they are determinedly open with both colleagues and patients. 'We trade in information, so there has to be a free flow—and that should include patients too,' Professor Marcus Pembrey, the department head believes.

The doctors' concern for their patients is almost tangible. The senior registrar reports 'a very tense situation' with a girl, 19-weeks pregnant, whose boyfriend has just confessed that his family has an inherited mental disorder. The girl says the boy has misled her; the boy's sister is on the phone to the doctor every day lobbying for her brother. Everyone agrees that the couple need time and careful counselling. They have an appointment at 1.45pm that day; happily, they can be told that only 10 per cent of children born with neurofibromatosis will have learning difficulties.

Then they discuss a batch of young women with a family history of genetic disorders who have applied for DNA testing to see if they are carriers of three common genetic diseases: cystic fibrosis, which clogs the lungs; muscular dystrophy, a wasting disease that affects boys only; and fragile X, increasingly recognised as a cause of mental impairment.

Many of the women are very young—the teenage sisters and cousins of sufferers. Once a directly inherited condition is identified, extended family screening and counselling are provided for those affected.

The final case demands detective work. The mother of a baby who died of respiratory failure and who was worryingly floppy at birth, is pregnant again. A ripple of concern runs round the room. The consensus is that there is a fairly high risk of recurrence. The doctors suggest that both mother and foetus should have tests and that investigations should be launched to locate the original paediatric records and to see if cells from the dead baby have been frozen for analysis.

Similar scenes are repeated at each of the 14 regional genetic centres throughout the country, which can be contacted direct by people anxious about their genetic inheritance. The genetics department at Great Ormond Street serves the Northeast Thames region and, though most patients are referred by their family doctors, anyone in the catchment area concerned about their history can ring and will, Professor Pembrey assures me, receive 'a friendly reception from the hospital'.

Despite the inevitable anxiety, the majority go away with the good news that there is little risk. But what happens when a genetic defect is identified?

Andrew Walker's greatest gift is his ability to show love and affection, says his mother Lesley. But though Andrew is 7, he has not yet outgrown the temper tantrums that can bring the local supermarket to an appalled standstill.

Andrew suffers from fragile X, which affects his ability to understand the world around him. At birth, he was smaller than his twin sister, and while Claire developed normally, Andrew was markedly slow. At nine months, his parents stopped pretending that 'boys are always behind', but it took nearly two years of tests, with the support of a determined consultant paediatrician, to establish the confused little boy's real problem.

Today, Andrew, who is severely affected and has an academic age of 2½, is becoming more manageable. One of his biggest problems is communication. Most words are just sounds that mean nothing to him, but there was a breakthrough recently when he started to say 'bye-bye' as he leaves for special school. But Lesley questions what life is like for Andrew, imprisoned in his own mind, and says she will never completely recover from the sense of guilt she felt when she heard the diagnosis. 'I was the carrier of the gene. I was the cause.'

Five years ago, when Lesley founded the Fragile X Support Group, she knew of only ten cases in the country; today it's believed that one child in 1000 inherits the condition. The discovery of the fragile X gene in May last year has revolutionised carrier testing. Although many cases are still undiagnosed (some doctors take the line, 'Why do you want to know when there's no cure?'), many can now be picked up by testing a single blood sample. Sufferers and their families should then be given the expert support and resources they need. And crucially, the possibility of pre-natal testing now allows prospective parents the choice Lesley was denied.

Because knowledge of genetics is so limited, many women are unaware that they're at risk. Despite the desirability of early counselling, many are first seen when they are already pregnant, and though DNA tests can now be carried out at ten weeks, leaving plenty of time for a termination, the emotional considerations are far from simple. Professor Pembrey confesses that his heart sinks when he is faced with a pregnant woman who is suspected of carrying a faulty gene. 'We might be able to do so much more to help if we only had time to sort it out.'

Not all conditions are as serious as fragile X, but the number means it's important that families should start compiling their own medical family tree. This can be started at any time, but Professor Pembrey suggests that a good time is when a couple get engaged or move in together, 'so relatives can see there is a reason for what may be called prying'.

Professor Pembrey also tends to encourage GPs to suggest patients investigate family health records. 'In the past, GPs quailed at the process, because if you found something, there was nothing to be done. Now the solution is referral to a genetic centre to sort out the problem.'

Compiling your health history

● Using our record sheet on page 211, fill in details of family members' illnesses, particularly those experienced under the age of 50. Note any disabilities (if the family member was thought 'backward', had epilepsy, was confined to a wheelchair or suffered unusual weakness), miscarriages and infant deaths.

● List details of every family member—great aunts and uncles, first cousins, blood-relatives' children from previous marriages—on a separate sheet of paper if necessary.

● Go back to your grandparents' generation at least—further if you can. (There was no history of fragile X for three generations in Lesley Walker's family and the inherited problem only became evident when her son was born.)

● File with your personal details (see page 212) and medical records of your own family.

Although you cannot change your genetic make-up, keeping a medical history can warn you of risks and may facilitate early diagnosis and suitable treatment.

How genes work

● You have 23 pairs of chromosomes made from strands of DNA incorporating 100,000 different genes. The genes carry the instructions for making each cell in your body.

● Genes are inherited, 50 per cent from your mother, 50 per cent from your father. If one gene alone can produce an effect it is dominant (like that for brown eyes). If a double dose is required, it is recessive (like the gene for blue eyes).

● Genetic diseases are caused by mutations, or damage to a gene. If a disease is caused by a recessive gene, a child has a 25 per cent chance of being affected, but only if both parents carry the defect. Genes can also be damaged in life if mistakes are made when cells divide and renew as part of the human growth process.

● Conditions such as haemophilia and muscular dystrophy are gender-linked, affecting males but carried by females.

Alan Havsteen-Mikkelsen was 50 and the father of five young children when he had a massive heart attack that destroyed 30 per cent of his heart muscle function. At the time, he was a heavy smoker, drinker and meat-eater, and as the head of a busy firm of architects, under relentless pressure. But though his lifestyle made his heart attack more likely, Professor Steve Humphries of University College Hospital says that when a coronary patient is under 55, there is a likelihood that genetic fac-

tors, as well as harmful habits such as smoking, are to blame. Alan's mother had died of a heart attack.

The prime suspect in Alan's case was thought to be genetic tendency to high cholesterol, which doctors say affects about one in 500 people.

The good news is that Alan's children will not inevitably be affected, even if they have inherited his vulnerability. It has become clear that a low-fat, high-fibre diet, plus exercise, stress management, giving up smoking and reducing alcohol consumption, have a strong, preventive effect. Alan is now a passionate supporter of a healthy, holistic lifestyle and his doctors are impressed with the progress he is making.

It's now clear that between 4,000 and 5,000 disease conditions are inherited. Currently, scientists are collaborating on the worldwide Human Genome Project, to produce a genetic 'road map' of the human body. This should be almost complete by the end of the century, if current disputes about the ethics of patenting sections of DNA where crucial genes are thought to lie are resolved.

So far, the project has located the exact position of about 50 disease genes, including haemophilia, sickle-cell anaemia, cystic fibrosis, muscular dystrophy, and severe combined immunodeficiency (ADA syndrome). The major ones outstanding now are the genes for the degenerative disease Huntington's chorea, and polycystic kidney disease.

Although technology enables scientists to map genes more rapidly than ever, academic knowledge outstrips practical application. DNA tests are available for some 50 conditions, but they are restricted to families known to be at risk—who live with the knowledge that there is, as yet, no sure way to prevent genetic illness, and no cure.

Despite this, future prospects are bright. Testing is already being carried out on embryos after in vitro fertilisation. This 'pre-implantation' screening is still at research stage, but a world first was achieved in March, when a healthy baby was born to a couple who each carry the cystic fibrosis gene. This has paved the way, says Professor Robert Winston at Hammersmith Hospital, whose team achieved the breakthrough, for similar screening for other single-gene defects.

Where treatment is concerned, hopes lie with gene therapy, where defective genes are replaced by healthy ones. Though still in its early stages, it's the first step to a possible cure.

Scientists have also discovered that inheriting a predisposition doesn't mean that illness is inevitable. 'The latest research suggests that many illnesses are the result of a complex interaction between a person's genetic predisposition and their environment,' says Professor Martin Bobrow of Guy's. Experts now believe many conditions fall into this category, including many types of cancer, heart disease, diabetes, allergies (including asthma and eczema), dyslexia, glaucoma and alcoholism.

Your mother should know

Sorting myth from fact in your family's health history can be difficult. Here are some of the statements you'll need to probe to establish the true picture.

● 'There was another baby, but it died at birth.' Was this a stillbirth or was there another cause?

● 'He/she was eccentric/hated meeting people.' Mental illness may not have been understood, or might have been thought shameful.

● 'He/she liked a drink/had a dreadful temper/was unpredictable.' The problem of alcoholism was (and still is) often underplayed.

● 'He/she was slow on the uptake/didn't go to school.' Learning difficulties (mental handicap) were hidden if possible.

● 'He/she had funny turns.' Was this epilepsy? It might also refer to Alzheimer's disease.

● 'Grandma/grandpa was chairbound by the time I was born.' The cause could be stroke, heart disease or a degenerative condition such as Parkinson's or motor neurone disease.

● 'I never knew my grandmother/father.' Check if they died from cancer or heart disease before 50.

● 'He/she had terrible skin problems/headaches/indigestion/sneezed all the time.' Is there a long-standing family history of allergy?

● 'He/she was very stooped/had trouble getting around.' Problems like this could be congenital or a sign of arthritis/osteoporosis in later life.

Cancers are probably the biggest group of life-threatening conditions now known to have a strong genetic component. Scientists have already located a gene for colon cancer, inherited by 1 per cent of each year's 27,500 new colon cancer patients—other genes are thought to be involved in a further 5–10 per cent of cases.

But experts such as Dr Roger Leicester at St George's Hospital, Tooting, believe that it's possible to reduce radically the 19,000 deaths every year. 'If we can identify and screen anyone with a positive family history really early on (ideally from

the age of 35) and remove any precancerous polyps, there is a 90 per cent-plus chance of cure,' he says.

The next revelation is likely to be the gene for early-onset breast cancer, known to be somewhere on the long arm of chromosome 17. Breast cancer is usually a disease of old age, and early development may be linked to a family history of the disease. Linda McGilvray was only 30 when cancer forced her to have a mastectomy. She wrote goodbye letters to her children and planned her funeral. But despite a second mastectomy, 12 years later, Linda is very much alive.

Because of her young age, the doctors suspected she had inherited a genetic predisposition to breast cancer. Linda had been adopted, and spent many hours researching at St Catherine's House until she found that her birth-mother and aunt had died of breast cancer relatively young.

Linda has now warned her 13-year-old daughter Kerry that she may have inherited a susceptibility to the illness, and a close watch will be kept on her.

But because it almost certainly takes several environmental triggers to activate the gene, many doctors believe there's a possibility of preventing the disease. There's evidence that a diet high in fruit, vegetables and fibre, low in saturated fats and alcohol, plus regular exercise and lower stress levels, can help protect against cancer as well as heart disease.

A more clinical approach is shown by the controversial tamoxifen trial, where high-risk women have volunteered to see if the drug can keep them cancer-free. It has proved very successful in the treatment of breast cancer, but critics, such as Dr Richard Nicholson of the Bulletin for Medical Ethics, argue that a drug known to have severe side-effects shouldn't be given to healthy women.

Although only a minority of cancers are thought to be directly linked to heredity, mapping the faulty genes in cancer, and indeed in all diseases, is vital, according to Dr Nigel Spurr of the Imperial Cancer Research Fund: 'Once we've worked out what they are doing, we should be able to block their activity or correct it, either with drugs or some other therapy.'

Ultimately the aim is to prevent genetically-linked illness, including many of the debilitating diseases of ageing. But Dr Spurr warns: 'We want to increase the quality of life, but that doesn't mean you can live forever. You can't change the course of nature.' What you can do is respect your genetic inheritance and design your life so it works for – not against – you.

Further information

- Contact-a-Family, 16 Strutton Ground, London SW1P 2HP (071-222 2695).

- The Genetic Interest Group, Institute of Molecular Medicine, John Radcliffe Hospital, Headington, Oxon OX3 9DU (0865 744002).

RESOURCE 5

Mange & Mange, Genetics: Human Aspects, 2nd Ed. 1990, p112–113

Nondisjunction of human autosomes: sporadic Down syndrome

One year after Mendel's work was published, the English physician John Langdon Down wrote a paper entitled 'Observations on an Ethnic Classification of Idiots'. As medical superintendent of an asylum for the severely retarded, he noted that about 10 per cent of all the inmates resembled each other and could be readily distinguished from the rest of the patients: 'So marked is this, that when placed side to side, it is difficult to believe that the specimens compared are not children of the same parents'. Because they had broad faces and slanted eyelids, he assumed they were 'typical Mongols', which we now know to be completely false.[1] Thus, what used to called 'mongolism' is now called Down syndrome. (A syndrome is a group of signs and symptoms that occur together and characterise a particular abnormality. Not all symptoms necessarily appear in every individual, however.)

General features

In addition to being retarded, Down syndrome patients exhibit some combination of the following traits which may vary considerably from one individual to another. All parts of the body are shortened, signifying poor skeletal development. The face is broad and flat with a small nose, irregular teeth, and abnormally shaped ears. The eyes may be close-set with narrow, slanting eyelids; a large, furrowed tongue may protrude from a mouth framed by rather thick lips. Hip bones are abnormally shaped and aligned, and the feet often display a sizeable gap between the first and second toes; the little finger is often short and curved inward. Some highly unusual patterns of hand creases plus hand and foot prints are also associated with Down syndrome – but with the advent of chromosome banding techniques, karyotope analysis has replaced dermatoglyphic (Greek derma, 'skin'; glyph, 'carving') analysis as a diagnostic tool. Nevertheless, attention to dermal patterns (along with other phenotypic traits) can, in the case of certain chromosomal disorders, alert physicians to the need for karyotype studies (Uchida and Soltan 1975).

Weak reflexes, loose joints, and poor muscle tone render these patients rather limp and floppy. Defects of the heart, digestive tract, kidneys, thyroid gland, and adrenal glands are also common. Males have poorly developed genitalia and are invariably sterile; in females, ovarian defects and irregular menstruation are the rule. Many Down syndrome babies die within a year, often from heart defects that occur in 40–50 per cent of them. Susceptibility to infection (especially pneumonia) is also common, probably due to defects in the immune system – but antibiotics and other medical improvements have extended the mean life expectancy to over 30 years, with 25 per cent of affected individuals surviving to the age of 50. Leukaemia is 15–20 times more frequent in Down syndrome patients than in the general population, and other types of cancer are more common too.

Motor development is slow, and bladder and bowel control may take years to develop. Many patients learn to talk, but speech is usually thick and harsh sounding, perhaps in part because of hearing defects. Lively, cheerful and very affectionate, Down syndrome patients are noted for their impishness, flair for mimicry, and enjoyment of music and dance. Although clumsy with their hands, they respond well to early intensive stimulation and training for simple tasks; despite IQs that seldom exceed 60, some learn to read and can attend regular classes.

Roughly 1–2 per cent of all live-born Down syndrome cases are mosaics, possessing both normal and abnormal cells. Not surprisingly, these individuals show great phenotypic variability in all respects – presumably depending upon the proportion and tissue location of the abnormal cells.

Possible relation to Alzheimer's disease

Ironically, delayed development is usually followed by premature ageing – often including, among those who survive beyond 30 years, dementia[2] of the type suffered by people with Alzheimer's disease. Indeed, recent neuropathological studies have uncovered some striking similarities in the brain abnormalities asociated with these two conditions.

References

[1]Down also suggested that 'the observations which I have recorded are indications that the differences in the races are not specific but variable. These examples of the result of degeneracy among mankind ... furnish some arguments in favour of the unity of the human species'. On these grounds he vigorously opposed slavery. He also supported higher education for women, denying that it would increase the risk of their producing feeble-minded children, a popular concern of the day.

[2]Memory loss, confusion, anxiety, loss of ability to perform simple tasks like dressing or feeding themselves, and ultimately the loss of all functional capabilities.

'Vaccine' hope for malignant melanoma

RESOURCE 6

Saul H, 'Gene therapy plan targets melanoma', New Scientist 1992, 135, 1840, 7; Nursing Standard, 14 October 1992

A 'simple' gene therapy to treat melanoma could begin clinical trials in Britain next year.

Although trying to find a gene that will 'turn off' cancer cells is the ultimate goal, researchers from St George's Hospital in London believe a simpler technique may be better in the short term. They have concentrated on boosting the immune response.

A protein called MHC Class I is usually vital to trigger the immune response to foreign proteins. Although cancer cells are not foreign, they are abnormal and are sometimes attacked. Melanoma cells lack MHC Class I and, therefore, go unrecognised. Using the protein as a 'vaccine' may alert the immune system to the cells. Animal experiments have been encouraging. It is unlikely the 'vaccine' will work on its own: it will probably be used after surgery to reduce the spread of malignant cells.

Vehicle pollutants: effects on the lung

RESOURCE 7

Stevan Monkley-Poole, Nursing Standard, 21 October 1992, Vol 7 No 5

As concern about pollution of the environment and the consequent effects on health grows nationally and internationally, the role of the nurse as health promoter is increasing in importance. The Royal College of Nursing responded to this concern by establishing an Environmental Working Party, of which the author is a member. This article considers one type of pollution, that caused by vehicles, and its effects on the functioning of the lung. The author argues that nurses need to be familiar with environmental determinants of health if they are to work towards upholding a 'health' service.

Air pollution is caused by a wide variety of human and natural sources. It is not a new phenomenon; London was regularly polluted by smogs for more than 100 years because the burning of coal releases sulphur dioxide emissions and particulates into the atmosphere.

In the infamous smog of 1952, an estimated 4,000 people died prematurely from exposure to high levels of air pollution (1). Today, it is the use of motor vehicles which, overall, produces more air pollution than any other single human activity (2). This article looks at the anatomy of the lungs and the effects of four major pollutants, sulphur dioxide, oxides of nitrogen, ozone and particulates, on the functioning of that organ. The article is not intended to be definitive and is offered as an introduction to the potential for damage of these ubiquitous substances.

Anatomy and defences

Unlike the quality of water, the benefits of cleaner air cannot be neatly categorised according to use. Air pollution, however, is recognised as being harmful to health (3, 4, 5).

The anatomy of the respiratory system

can be divided into three regions (*Figure 1*):

- Nasal, comprising the nose and mouth cavities and throat
- Tracheobronchial, beginning at the trachea and extending through the bronchial tubes to the alveolar sacs
- Pulmonary, comprising the terminal bronchi and the alveolar sacs, where gas exchange with the circulatory system occurs.

The trachea is about 10–11cm long and 2cm in mean diameter. At its lower end it divides into two main bronchi, left and right, one to each lung. The main bronchi divide into smaller bronchi up to a total of 11 branchings. Bronchioles are created by the divisions from 12th to the 16th.

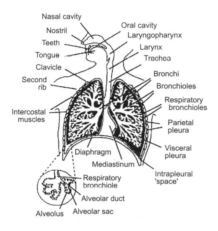

Figure 1 Anatomy of the respiratory system

The division process continues, culminating in alveolar ducts, alveolar sacs and the alveoli themselves. The portion of lung supplied by a terminal bronchiole is called an acinus, the basic functional unit of lung tissue. The ultimate area presented to the inspired air by these delicate walls of the millions of alveoli in each lung amounts to between 70 and 90 square metres.

Particles in the atmosphere, including vehicle emissions, may render the lungs vulnerable to a vicious circle of recurrent infection and damage to the tissues involved.

Air entering the respiratory passages is filtered by hairs and mucus in the nose. The trachea and larger bronchi are lined by cells, each of which contain a cilium. The cilia beat with a constant and coordinated motion.

This, in conjunction with mucus produced by cells in the wall of the trachea and bronchi, creates a 'self-cleaning' mechanism, a 'mucociliary escalator'. This traps fine particles which escape the nasal filter and carries them out of the respiratory tract. The mucus is either swallowed or expectorated (*Table 1*).

As inspired air passes down the trachea during inhalation, a vortex is created which tends to throw particles so that they fall upon and are trapped by the ciliary escalator (7).

There is a relationship between the aerodynamic size of particles and the regions where they are deposited. Larger particles are deposited in the nasal region by impaction on the hairs of the nose or at the bends of the nasal passages. Smaller particles pass through the nasal region and are deposited in the tracheobronchial and pulmonary regions.

Particles are removed by impacting with the walls of the bronchi when they are unable to follow the gaseous streamline flow through the subsequent bifurcations of the bronchial tree. As airflow decreases near the terminal bronchi, the smallest particles are removed by Brownian motion (oscillatory movement of particles resulting from bombardment by molecules moving at high velocity), which pushes them to the alveolar membrane (8).

In the pulmonary region, foreign particles can move across the epithelial lining of the alveolar sac to the lymph or blood systems, or they may be engulfed by alveolar macrophages. The macrophages can move to the mucociliary escalator for removal.

Inhaled particles in the atmosphere can range in size from less than 0.01 micrometres (μm) to more than 50 μm in diameter (8, 9). Dust, smoke and fumes contain particles which are capable of penetrating into the lung tissue. Dust particles range in size from a diameter of 1 μm to about 150 μm. Fumes are in the range of 0.2 μm to 1 μm. Industrial fumes often consist of oxides formed from hot or burning metals. Smoke has particles less than 0.3 μm in diameter.

These definitions are only a general indication of the relative sizes and are by no means absolute. Normally, only particles of a diameter less than 10 μm will float in the air for any length of time. It is those particles less than 5 μm which are likely to penetrate the defences of the lungs.

Bacteria and viruses are well within the limits allowing penetration of the respiratory tract, the average diameter ranging from 0.03 μm for smallpox and chickenpox (10). Those which enter are destroyed by the normal protective mechanisms. Any accumulation debris or liquid in the lungs is, however, likely to provide a focus for growth of opportunistic invaders. Local damage of tissue, obstruction of normal air flow, or failure to drain the lung of secretions adequately are therefore liable to encourage the development of localised infections. These may set up a vicious circle of recurrent infection and damage to the tissues involved.

Table 1 Clearance mechanism for removing foreign particles from the lungs (6)

- Rapid uptake of material deposited in the nasopharynx directly into the bloodstream.
- Rapid clearance of all particulate matter from the nasopharynx by ciliary transport of mucus.
- Rapid absorption of particles deposited in the tracheobronchial compartment into the systemic circulation.
- Rapid ciliary clearance of the tracheobronchial compartment. Particles cleared by this route go to the gastrointestinal tract.
- The direct translocation of material from the pulmonary region to the blood.
- The relatively rapid clearance phase of the pulmonary region dependent on recruitable macrophages. This in turn is coupled to the ciliary mucus transport process.
- A secondary pulmonary clearance process, dependent upon endocytosis and ciliary mucus transport.
- The slow removal of particles from the pulmonary compartment via the lymphatic system.
- The collective absorption of cleared material from the gastrointestinal tract into the blood.

Pollutants

Sulphur dioxide is the oldest known harmful air pollutant. Fossil fuels are sulphur rich and the sulphur is released when the fuel is burnt. Recent attention to damage caused by photochemical oxidants has tended to obscure the consequences to human health of this acidic gas (11). The worst damage from sulphur dioxide is associated with its role as precursor in sulphate formation (8). Sulphur dioxide is formed at a ratio of about 25–30 parts to one part sulphur trioxide, which then converts to atmospheric sulphuric acid in the presence of water vapour (1, 2).

Sulphate 'aerosols' are formed which are suspensions of colloidal ('gluelike') particles in a gas, compounded from sulphur trioxide and other basic oxides. Five to 20 per cent of total suspended particulate matter (TSP) is accounted for by these compounds, plus sulphuric acid mist.

Koenig and Pierson (4) point to sulphur dioxide causing a dramatic decrease in forced expiratory volume in one second. They also quote earlier studies showing increases in nasal airway resistance after exposure.

Another health effect attributed to the various sulphur oxides and sulphates is based on their irritant properties, because of the formation of sulphuric acid when sulphur trioxide combines with moisture in the lung. Particulates containing sulphates less than 1 mm in size cause most irritation. Larger particles may induce an involuntary coughing reflex.

Ninety per cent of inhaled sulphur dioxide is absorbed in the airways above the larynx. During severe short-term exposure, the negative ions (anions) of sulphate and sulphite formed on the moist cell surfaces of the nasal linings penetrate the mucosal cells and bind to granules within mast cells. This results in local release of histamine which acts as a local modulator to cause constriction of the airways and initiate local inflammation response. The acid mist is also thought to affect the ability to clear particles deposited in the small- and medium-sized airways (1).

Human tissues have the capacity to deal with bisulphate or sulphate through the activity of the enzyme sulphite oxidase. It has been calculated that a man breathing 5 parts per million (ppm) sulphur dioxide for eight hours would take up the equivalent of 1.3 mmol of bisulphate and sulphate during the day (11) (*Table 2*).

The lungs have apparently the capacity to remove more than 100 times this volume of sulphite oxidase. Calculations, however, are often spread over a whole day and throughout the whole lung. It is possible that intense confined accumulations in the epithelial tissues cannot be removed quickly enough before adverse localised damage occurs.

Oxides of nitrogen oxide and nitric

Table 2 Human response to different levels of sulphur dioxide (11)

Concentration (ppm)*	Period	Effects
0.03–0.5	Continuous	Condition of bronchitic patients worsened
0.3–1.0	20sec	Brain activity changed
0.5–1.4	1min	Odour perceived
1.3–1.5	15min	Increased eye sensitivity
1.0–5.0	30min	Increased lung airway resistance, sense of smell lost
1.6–5.0	<6hours	Constriction of nasal and lung passages
5.0–20.0	>6hours	Lung damage, reversible if exposure ceases
>20.0	>6hours	Waterlogging of lung passages and tissues, eventually leading to paralysis and/or death

*Generally lower if aerosols, particulate or other pollutants are also present oxide are the two most significant air pollutants (12). They are often referred to as total oxides of nitrogen. Formation occurs when combustion of fuels and certain chemical manufacturing operations take place.

Research studies, largely into nitrogen dioxide, to determine a model for the human situation and assess both the short and long term consequences from exposure, give a wide range of results. Some salient features do emerge, however.

Many factors are involved in the penetration and retention of oxides of nitrogen. The concentration in the air taken in, their reactivity, the length of exposure and the depth and frequency of breathing are all important factors relating to tissue fluids.

Because of its solubility, nitrogen dioxide will readily enter tissue fluid (mainly as nitrate). Similarly, nitric oxide may potentially enter, with more difficulty, as a mixture of nitrate and undissociated nitrous acid. The nasal regions, the terminal bronchioles, and finally the alveolar parenchyma therefore all have their surfaces exposed to the products of the oxides of nitrogen. Forty per cent of total oxides of nitrogen are taken up in the nose and throat regions during light breathing. When exercise is taken the balance shifts towards the most important uptake surfaces.

Low concentrations affect the areas of the junctions between the bronchioles and the alveolar regions. Ciliary cells and squamous surface cells may also be damaged. Higher concentrations extend the damage to the larger airways and into the deeper tissues.

Other changes include the formation of oedema, cellular debris or mucus and an aggregation of macrophages which accumulate as a natural line of defence against infection. Low concentrations of nitrogen dioxide have been shown to disturb the normal functioning of this process in animals.

The affinity of haemoglobin for absorbing nitrogen dioxide is 30,000 times greater than for oxygen and therefore will drastically reduce the carrying capacity (12).

Wellburn (11) suggests the presence of nitrogen oxide causes the haem of the red blood cells to form a type of methaemoglobin by chelation mechanisms, in which a metallic ion is sequestered and firmly bound into a ring within the chelating molecule. Some authors suggest that during short-term exposure to nitrogen dioxide, inflammation of lungs and bronchi occurs at 1.0ppm to 0.3ppm (9, 13).

Ozone reacts with almost every type of biological substance and is a powerful oxidising agent (1). Biological tissues and their close proximity to water lead to the formation of hydrogen peroxide and aldehydes by the process of 'ozonolysis'.

Ozone and its products disrupt membranes and the cellular functions dependent upon membranes by attacking the protein of those membranes. This is due to sensitivity of individual proteins on both the inside and outside of the cell, such as the transmembrane protein glycophorin. Levels need to be much higher before lipids are affected.

At low concentrations, ozone, like other photochemical oxidants, irritates the mucous membrane causing coughing, choking and impaired lung function through injury to the bronchiolar and alveolar walls. Surface epithelial cells which are damaged or destroyed are replaced by thick cuboidal cells with few cilia, thus reducing the effectiveness of the ciliary escalator. Oedema may accompany this initial damage and these symptoms may result in an acute inflammatory response. Epithelial cell ultrastructure may undergo change during such incidents leading to loss of cilia, cytoplasmic vacuolation and condensation of mitochondria into larger structures with abnormal cristae. It is reported that ozone interferes with the functions of lysozomes causing them to leak and prematurely ingest the host alveolar macrophage (11).

Similarly, ozone may cause macrophages to congregate and behave as if responding to a bacterial presence. If they become disabled due to their exposure to ozone, this leaves the lung tissue undefended against bacterial and viral assault.

Holman (1) claims there has been no systematic study into the effects of ozone on human health in the UK. Studies in America have recently shown it affects lung function at levels below the US National Ambient Air Quality Standard. Healthy men exposed to 240 μm/m^3 (about 120 parts per billion [ppb]) for nearly seven hours had difficulty breathing. Lung function decreased by 12 per cent. Difficulties continued even when doses were dropped to 80ppb.

Koenig and Pierson (4) propose that ozone causes a gradual decrease in pulmonary function which, unlike sulphur dioxide, persists for several hours. This is often accompanied by pain, making it difficult to inhale to total lung capacity.

Particulates

Particulates in the air consist of very small solid or liquid suspended droplets made up of many different substances. These may be within the range of 0.003μm to 500μm in diameter. Diesel vehicles, for example, emit black, fine oily particles in their exhaust and are of particular concern (3).

Complex organic compounds, such as

polyaromatic hydrocarbons, polycyclic organic matter and heavy metals are carried into the lungs on these particles.

An Organisation for Economic Cooperation and Development report (3) identifies a pilot study which suggests the risk ratio for the development of respiratory cancer was 42 per cent greater for those subjects exposed to diesel exhaust compared with those who were not. Godlee (5) reports that the International Air Agency for Research on Cancer concluded in 1988 that diesel engine exhaust is 'probably' carcinogenic to humans, and offers more supporting research for this view.

The small size of the particulates means they penetrate deeply into the pulmonary area of the lungs, which offer a large surface area for absorption of these carcinogenic, toxic and mutagenic compounds (3). Holman (1) suggests that particulates may have a synergistic effect with tobacco smoke, increasing the incidence of cancer above that expected from smoking alone.

Little doubt

It is important to acknowledge that there are problems with all the research based on human subjects. Our advanced industrial society, with its reliance on the internal combustion engine and concomitant exhaust fumes, ensures there is no such thing as an unexposed group.

Concentrations of air pollutants will vary depending on the location, and within those locations will be dependent upon factors such as weather conditions. Despite these factors, there can be little doubt that direct links can be shown between the compounds contained in exhaust fumes and damage to tissues.

This has implications for healthy subjects but more so for those people who are sensitive because of age, condition (such as pregnancy) or disease entity (asthma, bronchitis) (1, 2).

This article has looked at the effects of compounds in isolation. Some authors suggest, quite realistically, that the damaging effects are enhanced as the pollutants interact synergistically on the tissues exposed to them (2, 8).

Nurses and other health professionals spend a lot of time exhorting their patients/clients to adopt healthier life styles and habits. I have pointed to areas that have important implications for health and yet seem beyond people's immediate control. Environmental determinants of health encompass both the life-sustaining elements whose sufficiency needs to be assured and the life threatening elements whose sufficiency needs to be contained. Nurses need to be familiar with both, to be able to work towards upholding a 'health' service.

References

1. Holman C. Air Pollution and Health. London, Friends of the Earth. 1989.

2. Read R, Read C. Breathing can be hazardous for your health. New Scientist. 1991. 129, 1757, 34–37.

3. Organisation for Economic Co-operation and Development. Transport and the Environment. France, OECD. 1988.

4. Koenig J Q, Pierson W E. Air pollutants and the respiratory system: toxicity and pharmacologic interventions. Clinical Toxicology. 1991. 29, 3, 401–411.

5. Godlee F. Air pollution II: road traffic and modern industry. British Medical Journal. 1991. 303, 1539–1543.

6. Purdom P W. Environmental Health. Second edition. London, Academic Press. 1980.

7. Rowland A J, Cooper P. Environment and Health. London, Edward Arnold. 1983.

8. Stern A C et al. Fundamentals of Air Pollution. London, Academic Press. 1984.

9. Tolley G S et al. Environmental Policy: Air Quality. Cambridge MA, Ballinger. 1982.

10. Cooke E M. Hare's Bacteriology and Immunology for Nurses. Seventh edition. Edinburgh, Churchill Livingstone. 1991.

11. Wellburn A. Air Pollution and Acid Rain. London, Longman Scientific and Technical. 1988.

12. Tewari A, Shukla N P. Air pollution: effects of nitrogen dioxide. Reviews on Environmental Health. 1989. 8, 1–4, 157–163.

13. Carlisle D. Air care. Nursing Standard. 1989. 3, 43, 20–21.

Stevan Monkley-Poole RMN, DPSN, is Lecturer, Normanby College of Health Care Studies, a member of the Environmental Working Party and co-opted member of the Health and Social Policy Committee of the Royal College of Nursing.

Radiant health?

RESOURCE 8

A Doctor Writes, by John Collee The Observer Magazine, 28 November 1992

If you drive through the Lake District and carry on down to the sea you will arrive at Seascale and, just along the coast, the Sellafield nuclear reactor. It was in 1983 that a Yorkshire Television documentary suggested that the incidence of childhood leukaemia in this area was higher than elsewhere. The Black Committee confirmed the programme's basic findings: leukaemia is so rare in children that the odds were 4:1 against finding even a single case in Seascale. In fact there were four.

One might have anticipated that this would be a death-blow to the nuclear industry, but the case against it has never been proven. Irradiation, as we know, has a weak but significant ability to cause cancer. Children are more readily affected than adults, and the cells of the marrow, in which leukaemia originates, are more radiosensitive than most tissues. On the other hand, co-existence doesn't imply causality. One might find a cluster of heart attacks near a brewery, but even if you were convinced that heart attacks are caused by the smell of hops, you would still have to acknowledge the possibility of other causes.

So British Nuclear Fuels argued, correctly, that further research was needed. To many this sounded like filibustering, but then came a report from the National Radiological Protection Board which showed that the external radiation from Sellafield amounted to only 16 per cent of the normal background radiation, and was therefore unlikely to be causing the 16-fold (1600 per cent) rise in childhood leukaemia at Seascale.

Unless, of course, the radiation was internal. Cancer can be caused by isotopes of, say, plutonium which are inhaled or eaten and are afterwards difficult to detect. Infants are particularly efficient at absorbing plutonium. Once absorbed, it concentrates in the bone and irradiates the marrow. Nuclear fuel reprocessing plants such as Sellafield produce plutonium.

Apart from Sellafield, one other plant in Britain undertakes nuclear fuel reprocessing: Dounreay in the far north of Scotland. In 1986 the Scottish Health Service mapped out its leukaemia data and found that one of the most impressive clusters was in Thurso, just down the coast from Dounreay. This looked like a decisive second-half goal to the anti-nuclear lobby.

Again the amount of exposure was calculated, again it was found to be insufficient to account for the level of cancers. This assumed of course that the stated level of emissions was accurate. A former Sellafield scientist called Dr Jakeman had already drawn attention to a past accident in which 20kg of uranium oxide was released. So if accidents had happened, was it not suspicious that all six of the Dounreay cases occurred in a five-year period between 1979 and 1984? Had there perhaps been a huge release of, say,

plutonium, which we didn't know about?

Plutonium is handled at military establishments concerned with nuclear weapons, such as the Atomic Weapons Research Establishment at Aldermaston and the Royal Ordnance factory at Burghfield. A paper published in 1987 reported an increase in childhood leukaemia around these two towns.

To the anti-nuclear lobby this confirmed the link between leukaemia and plutonium-handling establishments. Ironically, the Aldermaston-Burghfield cluster provided valuable ammunition for the opposition, because the feasible emissions from such a plant were so tiny that plutonium pollution couldn't possibly be the cause of the cancers.

British Nuclear Fuels received another fillip in 1989 when it was found that the incidence of leukaemia was increased in areas designated for nuclear installations which had not yet been built. This suggested that the cause of the leukaemia clusters were some non-nuclear factor common to those places where you would decide to build a nuclear installation – remoteness, proximity to the sea, certain rock structures and so on.

A variation on this theory, put forward by epidemiologist Leo Kinlen, was that leukaemia is caused by a virus. He argued that the influx of outsiders at nuclear establishments and elsewhere may expose the non-immune local population to this infection. This might explain the cluster of childhood leukaemias in Glenrothes, which grew in the 1950s from a village to a new town. But it doesn't explain Aldermaston, which was heavily populated long before they started making nuclear bombs there.

To further complicate things, the irradiation explanation has been put firmly back on the agenda by Professor Martin Gardner and his colleagues at Southampton. They have found that leukaemia and lymphoma are more likely in young people whose fathers received a large dose of radiation. Leukaemia, they argue, is in this case a reflection of inherited genetic damage and is therefore determined by the radiation dose to the parent working inside the factory.

Annoyingly, this explains some of the cases but not all of them. Do we ditch the genetic environmental and viral theories, or do we assume that all of them apply? Nobody knows. In the past nine years the only thing that has been proven beyond doubt is that it is better to be a documentary-maker than an epidemiologist. Documentary-makers only have to pose a difficult question. Epidemiologists have to solve the blasted thing.

Breast cancer treatment offers hope

RESOURCE 9A

Chris Milhill,
Medical Correspondent,
The Guardian,
5 June 1992

An experimental method of boosting the body's defence system using a series of injections may offer an avenue of hope for women with breast cancer, scientists said yesterday.

Researchers from the Imperial Cancer Research Fund stressed at a press conference in London that the approach – immunotherapy – was at an early stage, but it could open the way for a new class of anti-cancer treatment.

Breast cancer kills 15,700 women a year in the UK, while annually there are 25,000 new cases. It is the largest single killer of women in the South, although lung cancer has overtaken it in the North. Sixty-two per cent of patients survive for five years, but the earlier it is diagnosed the greater the chance of survival.

Joyce Taylor-Papadimitriou has discovered that a molecule called mucin is present in normal cells, but differs when it occurs in tumours. The cancerous version has far less sugar, but the body's immune system does not recognise this as sufficiently different to mount an attack on the cancer molecule. Dr Taylor-Papadimitriou, head of the ICRF's epithelial cell biology laboratory, has found a way of producing the abnormal molecule with its deficient sugar content in the laboratory.

It is hoped that injections of this will stimulate the body's own defence systems in a way that the naturally occurring substance does not, allowing the tumour to be attacked.

Dr David Miles, of Guy's Hospital, London, is to carry out a study of 40 women who have had relapses of breast cancer. Research in a handful of patients in Canada has shown that the approach is safe, and there is some evidence that tumours have shrunk.

Dr Taylor-Papadimitriou said: 'If we can do this successfully it would have a wide range of applications.' It was possible that the application early in the disease might have a preventive effect.

Dr Miles commented: 'It's a totally new approach and we have a lot to learn, but it opens up the prospect for new and perhaps more effective ways of treating breast cancer.'

The charity meanwhile needs £10 million for a new unit to speed up the transfer of laboratory knowledge about breast cancer into patient care.

Further Information

Saving More Lives, Public Relations Department, ICRF, PO Box 123, Lincoln's Inn Fields, London WC2A 3PX. £1.50 plus 9x12 SAE.

Geneticists make breakthrough in heart treatment

RESOURCE 9B

Robin McKie,
Science Correspondent,
The Observer,
25 October 1992

The world's first attempt to correct a genetic predisposition to heart disease appears to have succeeded. One of the team responsible for the breakthrough says she is now confident that it will lead to an improvement in the general treatment of coronary failure – the West's biggest killer.

Scientists at the Michigan University in Ann Arbor carried out the treatment in June, inserting genetically-altered liver cells into a 27-year-old French-Canadian who suffers from severe cholesterol build-up in her arteries. And last week, they reported that preliminary results were 'extremely encouraging'. The patient's liver had begun to manufacture life-saving cholesterol-absorbing chemicals.

Now the Michigan team plans two more revolutionary gene therapy treatments on patients with inherited heart disease this year, and a further 10 operations in 1993.

Eventually the team, led by Dr James Wilson, hopes it will be able to develop gene therapy techniques for a wide range of congenital heart conditions. 'So far results have been very encouraging,' said Dr Maryanne Grossman, a member of

Dr Wilson's team.

The condition tackled by the team is known as familial hypercholesterolaemia, and it comes in two forms. In the first type, patients lack a gene for a chemical known as the LDL receptor protein, whose function is to reduce cholesterol in the blood. Cholesterol, a basic nutritional requirement of the body, can build up in arteries causing heart disease. It is the function of the receptor to mop up any excess and prevent this.

Those who inherit an inoperative gene that should make the receptor protein – about one in 500 is affected – lack the power to break down cholesterol. However, as our genes come in pairs, there is usually a second receptor gene to make some of the 'mop-up' protein and scavenge some of the cholesterol in affected blood.

Nevertheless, their cholesterol levels are usually double the average, leaving them prone to heart attacks and coronary disease by the time they are in their late forties. Occasionally such individuals meet other victims, marry and have children. And occasionally such a child will inherit a malfunctioning gene from both parents. The accretion of cholesterol can produce symptoms in a six-year-old that is normally only seen in an adult who has smoked, drunk and eaten too much for decades.

Fortunately, the incidence of severe familial hypercholesterolaemia is very low. But doctors have difficulty helping these people because cholesterol-reducing drugs act by stimulating the receptor gene the children lack. The alternatives are a liver transplant from a matched donor, or complete blood transfusions every two or three weeks. Few victims live beyond the age of 30.

This is why the woman was treated by the team. It removed cells from her liver and infected them with a virus that had been genetically engineered to carry the protein gene she lacked.

The virus carried the gene into her chromosomes where it lodged, though the take-up rate was sporadic. The cells were returned to the patient, where they began to make small amounts of receptor protein.

The team, which has been inundated with letters from desperate parents of affected children, is working on methods for linking receptor genes to other chemicals absorbed by liver cells, to help victims of a milder form of the disease.

'We are going to learn so much about heart disease that there cannot fail to be an improvement in the general treatment of the West's biggest killer,' said Dr Grossman.

RESOURCE 9C

Nursing Standard No 27 Vol 6/32, 1992

Papillomavirus the key to cervical detection

The detection of underlying disease in women with slightly abnormal cervical smears may be increased through testing for evidence of human papillomavirus, according to a report in The Lancet.

Over five million cervical smears are examined in the UK each year, of which about 5 per cent show some abnormality. Severe dyskaryosis, usually indicative of high-grade cervical neoplasia, is found in about 10 per cent of abnormal smears.

The majority of abnormal smears show mild or moderate dyskaryosis, and the management of women with such smears is controversial, the report says. Its authors say a non-invasive test that accurately predicts which women have high-grade neoplasia would prove beneficial, and suggests that the detection of human papillomavirus type 16 (HPV 16) DNA in cervical smears would serve this purpose.

The report says that in almost 90 per cent of 85 women referred for colposcopy because of abnormal cytology, intermediate or high levels of HPV 16 predicted the presence of cervical cancer, irrespective of the cytological grade of the smear. The researchers say their findings indicate 'that colposcopic investigation of women with mild or moderate dyskaryosis is appropriate when increased amounts of HPV 16 DNA are also present'.

Gill Oliver, Chair of the RCN's Cancer Nursing Society, said the research was welcome if it helped indicate which women needed active treatment. 'Without that sort of information, we are not always certain who should have treatment and who should be watched,' she said.

Genetic gel could halt vessel occlusion

RESOURCE 9D

*Nursing Standard,
28 October 1992*

A gel which cancels genetic instructions could have beneficial effects in coronary artery disease.

American researchers have developed a gel which contains molecules specifically designed to block genetic function. If used after procedures such as balloon angioplasty, the gel might prevent re-occlusion.

Angioplasty causes damage to the vessel wall which the body tries to repair by producing smooth muscle cells. But this repair mechanism can lead to re-occlusion. The gel appears to interfere with the production of a protein which is essential to the process of smooth muscle cell formation.

So far, the gel has only been tried in animal models. It dried to a translucent film and appeared to prevent smooth muscle cells forming where it had been applied.

Alzheimer's disease: advances in genetics

RESOURCE 10

*Mary Wilde
Nursing Standard,
22 July 1992*

Recent advances in DNA technology have allowed identification of those carrying the gene mutation for early-onset Alzheimer's disease in some families, and provide the prospect of an effective treatment or cure in the future. While last week's article questioned the existence of late-onset Alzheimer's as a distinct disease entity, this one illustrates how and why these scientific advances may have far-reaching psycho-social consequences for some family members. It suggests why there is likely to be an increase in demand for the kind of information and support which can be offered by a genetic counselling service.

Alzheimer's disease (AD) is the commonest of the pre-senile dementias [1] and age-related cerebral disorders, with one in five people being affected by the eighth decade [2]. It is the largest single cause of dementia in elderly people: the widely-held view that senile dementia is most commonly the result of arteriosclerotic degeneration being incorrect [3].

AD is a neurodegenerative disorder with loss of memory, declining cognitive function, language disturbances, visiospatial disorientation, deterioration in social skills and motivation and, ultimately, deteriorating physical functioning proceeding to complete helplessness. Death usually occurs within three to seven years of the onset of symptoms and signs.

Although there is some overlap between the neurological changes in AD and those seen in the normal ageing brain, AD does not appear to be simply an exaggeration of the ageing process. A definite diagnosis requires pathological confirmation at autopsy, the characteristic neuropathological findings being abundant amyloid plaques, cerebrovascular amyloid and neurofibrillary tangles. Clinical diagnosis is more difficult and inaccuracy in diagnosis is estimated in about 10 per cent of cases [4].

Aetiology and genetic linkage

The aetiology of AD is poorly understood and there is no known treatment or cure. Effective treatment is, in fact, no nearer than when Alzheimer originally described the disorder in 1907 [5]. Rosser [6] estimated that in 1987 there were some 570,000 people in Britain suffering from AD.

Evidence has been presented to support the division of AD families into two distinct diagnostic groups, that is early onset (before the age of 65) and late onset (after 65) [7]. The early-onset group exhibits the expected 50 per cent risk of a dominantly inherited disorder (*Figure 1*), while the late-onset group shows offspring affected above the 50 per cent risk level, suggesting either non-Mendelian inheritance and/or the inclusion of non-genetic cases. Genetic studies suggest more than one underlying cause [8].

Evidence from genetic linkage studies (which demonstrate the presence of linkage between the gene locus for a particular disorder and an adjacent chromosomal segment, as shown by genetic markers), suggests that AD can be caused by a defect on a gene on the proximal long arm of chromosome 21 (*Figure 2*) in some early-onset families [9].

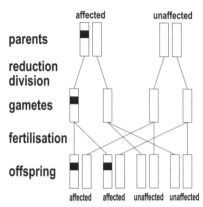

Figure 1 Showing possible outcomes at fertilisation in the mating between a person carrying the gene for an autosomal dominant disorder (black line) and a person not carrying the gene, resulting in a 50 per cent risk to offspring for each pregnancy.

Interest in searching for mutations of chromosome 21 began with the observation that the classical neuropathological and neurochemical changes found in AD invariably developed some ten to 30 years earlier in individuals with Down syndrome (trisomy 21) than in those without Down syndrome [10]. The proportion of cases with a genetic aetiology is unknown, but studies have consistently demonstrated that family history is a major risk factor for developing the disease [11].

Recent work by Goate et al [12] supports the hypothesis that genetic factors can influence the age at which an individual develops what many researchers believe will be an inevitable consequence of growing old.

A study of 39 members of a Nottingham-based family, where early-onset AD (confirmed by autopsy) was segregating in an autosomal dominant pattern, revealed a mutation within the amyloid precursor protein (APP) gene on the long arm of chromosome 21 in all affected individuals. The mutation was not found in any of the 200 chromosomes studied from unaffected individuals.

The same mutation was found in a second unrelated kindred with early-onset AD but was not demonstrated in other families studied. (Some other families now show this mutation but they are a tiny percentage of all AD families.) The conclusion drawn was that some cases of AD would be caused by mutations within the APP gene. How the mutation might lead to the characteristic neuropathological changes seen in AD has yet to be determined.

The finding has led to optimism that the actual gene locus for early-onset AD will be identified, the molecular basis for the neuropathological changes will be explained and, ultimately, an effective treatment or even a cure will be found. Telephone enquiries to the Nottingham Clinical Genetics Department from concerned relatives of affected people suggested that dissemination of the news by the non-scientific media led to the inevitable surge of false hopes about effective treatments or a cure.

Clinical application of research

While the work represents an important advance in the understanding of the aetiology of AD, it raises many implications for sufferers and their families and is likely to increase demands for the kind of help and support which can be offered by a genetic counselling service.

There is a wide variation in people's concepts of what genetic counselling involves. Harper [1] summarises the concept succinctly: '... Genetic counselling is the process by which patients or relatives at risk of a disorder that may be hereditary are advised of the consequences of the disorder, the probability of developing and transmitting it and the ways in which this may be prevented or ameliorated.'

As part of the counselling team, the nurse makes the initial contact with the family referred to the Clinical Genetics Service, carrying out an initial assessment of counselling needs and potential problems and exploring the family's expectations of the service. The initial meeting usually takes place in the family's home, where the nurse obtains and records pedigree information (essential if counselling is to be accurate) and explains how the service attempts to help those who find themselves in need of this type of care.

This home visit affords the opportunity for correcting misconceptions and for initiating counselling as appropriate. The nurse attends the counselling clinic with the family and assesses any follow-up needs, liaising with both professionals and lay groups to ensure that comprehensive support is available to facilitate adjustment to the burden of genetic disease, and retaining the family's link with the Genetic Service as further counselling needs arise and medical technological advances are made.

The counselling process is a two-way communication between the person being counselled and a genetic counselling team which has to be aware that the information communicated may be of a very personal and delicate nature in situations which may be '... emotionally charged with feelings of guilt and recrimination, frequently coupled with loss of self-

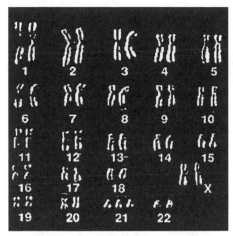

Figure 2 Interest in mutations of chromosome 21 began with the discovery that neuropathological changes found in AD often developed ten to 30 years earlier than usual in people with Down syndrome (trisomy 21).

esteem'. [13].

Many people who appear to have a dominant family history of AD have never in the past been given the opportunity to talk to a genetic counsellor and many may have suffered needlessly from misinformation and misconceptions about 'carriers' or 'skipped generations', and a truthful and factual explanation can do a great deal to relieve some of this suffering.

The individual's perceptions of AD will obviously depend upon previous experience and how involved the person has been in the direct care of affected family members. Advice from relatives and friends may have been particularly gloomy and intimidating and some may find it reassuring to hear that the risks are fewer than they believed.

Learning about dominant inheritance and the 50 per cent risk to offspring of affected individuals may equally be very traumatic for some people who have previously accepted what they saw to be an unfortunate coincidence in the family and who may be ill-prepared to cope alone with this new knowledge.

A young adult may be enraged with the parent who is 'responsible' for this risk, at the same time as being distraught by the 'loss of the person' loved as a parent. Those 'at risk' are often confronted by witnessing the gradual deterioration of a loved one's intellect and personal relationships, a constant reminder of exactly what one is 'at risk' from developing.

Persons receiving information about the inheritance of AD may be doing so while trying to cope with the emotional, physical, social and financial burdens of caring for an affected relative or while trying to achieve some balance between the competing pressures of goals and obligations, and living with the stigma which still prevails in relation to dementia. It is not the role of the counselling team to attempt to order the lives of others and genetic counselling should always be non-directive.

A major consequence of the scientific advances for the Nottingham family cited earlier, was that the genetic mutation could be easily identified from a blood sample, that is individuals now at 50 per cent risk of inheriting the condition from an affected parent could be offered a blood test which would show with 95 per cent accuracy whether or not they would develop the condition in the fifth decade. (In this family, the mean age of onset of symptoms in affected individuals was 57, all individuals developing symptoms between the ages of 52 and 61). The majority of those carrying the gene will have produced families before they succumb. In this way the disease has been transmitted through several generations.

Many individuals may not wish to avail themselves of a predictive presymptomatic test, but others may have found living with uncertainty intolerable and would welcome clarification of their status before making future domestic, reproductive and professional plans. Such testing raises both practical and ethical questions and must be preceded and followed by expert counselling, with thoughtful organisation of long-term support for those who receive a 'bad' result.

The availability of predictive testing may expose those 'at risk' to coercion by family, friends, employers, insurers, financial companies and even society in general, to undergo testing, and to the ultimate discrimination of 'positive' individuals, reinforcing ideas that they are genetically flawed. (Failure to divulge a 'positive' result from a presymptomatic test on insurance/mortgage proposals which specifically ask for this information will render the transaction invalid.)

In a free society, the decision to have children must always rest with individual couples, but couples belonging to AD families may find the decision less straightforward and may need help to cope with their reproductive choices. Such individuals may fear that they will be seen to be irresponsible if they choose to have children, finding the thought of years ahead of childlessness unbearable.

Many may feel that the risk is worth taking, in anticipation of major genetic advances being made over the next 50 years, leading to a cure or prevention of

AD. There may, of course, be pressure from family and friends to opt for predictive testing prior to making reproductive decisions or to explore the feasibility of pre-natal testing for potential offspring, with the aim of terminating those foetuses found to be carrying the genetic mutation.

Some couples may not wish to have individual genetic status clarified, but may wish to discuss the feasibility of ovum or sperm donation, in an attempt to ensure that there is no possibility of passing on the disease to the next generation.

Summary

This paper has concentrated on the author's experiences of the psychosocial sequelae realised by some members of early-onset AD families. Late-onset disease is by far the most common and there is some evidence to suggest that genetic factors play a part in its aetiology, with researchers proposing that absence of a Mendelian model of inheritance in a particular family may be due to the fact that individuals may have died from other causes before reaching the age at which they would develop clinical features of AD [11].

If this is so, then the situation should become clearer as the population shows greater longevity in forthcoming decades.

The work of the genetic counselling team has to be seen as only one part of the total care needed by families affected by familial AD, but it is hoped that as future developments in DNA technology provide insight into the precise aetiological mechanisms involved, the counselling service will continue to be available to provide information and support as families attempt to come to terms with the multiplicity of problems that both the disorder and scientific advances lay at their feet.

References

1. Harper P. Practical Genetic Counselling, London, Wright. 1988.

2. Mortimer et al, cited by Write A. Beta amyloid resurrected. Nature. 349, 653–654.

3. Wilcock G K. The challenge of Alzheimer's Disease – no longer a silent epidemic. Health Trends. 1988. 20, 17–19.

4. Haines J L. The genetics of Alzheimer Disease – a teasing problem. American Journal of Human Genetics. 1991. 48, 1021–1025.

5. Roberts G W. All quiet on the Southern Front. Journal of the Royal College of Physicians of London. 1988. 22, 2, 101–103.

6. Rosser M N. Dementia. British Journal of Hospital Medicine. 1987. 38, 47–50.

7. Farrer L A et al. Transmission and age-at-onset patterns in familial Alzheimer's Disease: evidence for heterogeneity. Neurology. 1990. 40, 395–403.

8. St George Hyslop P II et al. Genetic linkage studies suggest that Alzheimer's Disease is not a single homogeneous disorder. Nature. 1990. 194–197.

9. Goate A M et al. Predisposing locus for Alzheimer's Disease on chromosome 21. The Lancet. 1989. i, 352–355.

10. Lai F, Williams R S. A Prospective study of Alzheimer Disease in Down Syndrome. Archives of Neurology. 1989. 46, 849–853.

11. Breitner J C S. Clinical genetics and genetic counselling in Alzheimer Disease. Annals of Internal Medicine. 1991. 115, 8, 601–606.

12. Goate A M et al. Segregation of a missense mutation in the amyloid precursor protein gene with familial Alzheimer's Disease. Nature. 1991. 349, 704–706.

13. Emery A E H, Pullen I. Psychological Aspects of Genetic Counselling. London, Academic Press. 1984.

FURTHER READING

AGGLETON, P and CHALMERS, H (1984) *The Roy Adaptation Model*, Oxford, Blackwell.

BMA (1992) *Our Genetic Future: The Science and Ethics of Genetic Technology*, Oxford University Press.

CAMPBELL, J 'Making Sense of the Principles of Genetics', *Nursing Times* 88 (27) 36-38.

DAWSON, F M 'Sickle Cell Disease: Implications for Nursing Care', *Journal of Advanced Nursing*, 11 (6) 729-738.

FITZIMMONDS, J S A (1980) *Handbook of Clinical Genetics*, London, Heinemann.

ROY, C (1980) *Conceptual Models of Nursing Practice*, Norwalk CT Appleton Century Crafts.